AGELESS FITNESS

CRISTINA SEGREDO

Copyright © 2024 by Cristina Segredo.

All rights reserved. No part of this publication may be reproduced, distributed or transmitted in any form or by any means, electronic or mechanical, including photocopying, recording, or by any information storage and retrieval system, without permission in writing from the copyright owner, except in the case of brief quotations embodied in critical reviews and certain other noncommercial uses permitted by copyright law.

Although the author and publisher have made every effort to ensure that the information in this book was correct at press time, the author and publisher do not assume and hereby disclaim any liability to any party for any loss, damage, or disruption caused by errors or omissions, whether such errors or omissions result from negligence, accident, or any other cause.

Adherence to all applicable laws and regulations, including international, federal, state and local governing professional licensing, business practices, advertising, and all other aspects of doing business in the U.S., Canada, or any other jurisdiction is the sole responsibility of the reader and consumer.

Neither the author nor the publisher assumes any responsibility or liability whatsoever on behalf of the consumer or reader of this material. Any perceived slight of any individual or organization is purely unintentional.

The resources in this book should not be used to replace the specialized training and professional judgement of a healthcare professional.

Neither the author nor the publisher can be held responsible for the use of the information provided within this book. Please always consult a trained professional before making any decision regarding treatment of yourself or others.

eBook ASIN: B0D57GV91C
Paperback ISBN: 979-8-218-84354-0
Audiobook ISBN:

AGELESS FITNESS LIFESTYLE

Fitness and wellness are a lifestyle which start with your mindset. In every stage of life, one benefits from prioritizing their health and maintaining an active lifestyle. The benefits surpass aesthetics and physical appearance, transcending into deep-rooted inner peace, joy, and mental sharpness. An ageless fitness lifestyle is one of the most sacred and valuable commitments you can make to yourself. We wholeheartedly believe this lifestyle is an investment towards living a long-lasting, prosperous, high-quality life.

Our mission is to educate, empower, and guide anyone who is wanting and willing to work towards living their best ageless fitness lifestyle. We hope to provide a sense of hope and inspiration to everyone in an inclusive environment, where specific age and baseline fitness levels do not serve as barriers. Targeted towards older adults, but not limited to exact age or circumstances, our vision understands that everyone's body and journey are unique, and we aspire to impact positive change and meet you wherever you are in your process. A mustard seed of intention, motivation, and work can snowball into a complete lifestyle change with the right direction and influence.

Welcome to the ageless fitness movement. We hope you enjoy the ride!

This book is dedicated to my mom, dad, and their friends, with love, to encourage you to stay healthy and maintain the best quality of life as you retire and enter your golden years. May this guide help you to make them the best years yet!

TABLE OF CONTENTS

AGELESS FITNESS LIFESTYLE 3

About the Author 11

Introduction to Ageless Fitness 15
    1.1 The Importance of Fitness in Older Adults 15
    1.2 Benefits of Regular Exercise for Older Adults 18
    1.3 Overcoming Barriers to Fitness in Older Age 20
    1.4 Setting Realistic Fitness Goals for Older Adults 25

Fitness Guide for Older Adults 28
    2.1 Assessing Fitness Levels in Older Adults 28
    2.2 Designing a Safe and Effective Exercise Program 36
    2.3 Incorporating Strength Training for Older Adults 41
    2.4 Utilizing Balance and Stability Exercises for Seniors 42
    2.5 Implementing Low-Impact Cardio Workouts for Seniors 44
    2.6 Managing Joint Pain through Exercise for Seniors 45
    2.7 Enhancing Functional Training for Daily Activities in Older Age 47
    2.8 Improving Posture and Relieving Back Pain in Elderly Individuals 49

Strength Training for Older Adults..52
  3.1 The Benefits of Strength Training in Older Age 52
  3.2 Selecting Appropriate Resistance and Equipment..........55
  3.3 Upper Body Strength Exercises...58
  3.4 Lower Body Strength Exercises...61
  3.5 Core and Abdominal Strength Exercises............................64
  3.6 Designing a Well-Rounded Strength Training
       Routine 67

Balance and Stability Exercises 73
  4.1 The Importance of Balance and Stability in Older
       Age...73
  4.2 Assessing Balance and Stability Levels 75
  4.3 Balance Exercises into Daily Routine 80
  4.4 Stability Exercises to Improve Coordination......................82
  4.5 Core Strength for Better Balance and Stability................86

Low-Impact Cardio Workouts 90
  5.1 The Benefits of Low-Impact Cardio for Older
       Adults..90
  5.2 Choosing Suitable Cardio Exercises 92
  5.3 Cardio Workouts without Straining Joints.........................94
  5.4 Modifying Intensity and Duration of Cardio
       Workouts 97
  5.5 Creating a Varied and Enjoyable Cardio Routine.......... 101

Joint Pain Management Through Exercise 104
  6.1 Common Joint Pain Issues in Older Adults..................... 104
  6.2 The Role of Exercise in Managing Joint Pain.................. 107
  6.3 Incorporating Joint-Friendly Exercises into Fitness

Routine 109
6.4 Stretching and Flexibility Exercises for Joint Pain Relief 115
6.5 Using Proper Form and Technique to Prevent Joint Strain 119

Functional Training for Daily Activities 123
7.1 The Importance of Functional Training in Older Adults 123
7.2 Identifying Functional Fitness Goals for Daily Activities 126
7.3 Functional Exercises into Fitness Program 129
7.4 Improving Mobility and Range of Motion for Daily Tasks 135
7.5 Enhancing Strength and Endurance for Independent Living 140

Posture Improvement and Back Pain Relief 144
8.1 Understanding the Impact of Aging on Posture and Back Health 144
8.2 Assessing Posture and Identifying Areas of Improvement 148
8.3 Incorporating Posture-Correcting 155
8.4 Strengthening Core Muscles for Better Posture 158
8.5 Stretching and Mobility Exercises 161

Maintaining an Ageless Fitness Lifestyle 164
Adapting to Your Evolving Needs 164
Holistic Approach to Fitness 166
Living the Ageless Fitness Philosophy Daily 168

ABOUT THE AUTHOR

Cristina Segredo is a Doctor of Physical Therapy who has been dedicated to changing lives and molding minds in the healthcare and wellness field for over 15 years. As a physical therapist and fitness expert, she has a plethora of experience in the realm of rehabilitating neurologic and orthopedic injuries, as well as a background in exercise science and personal training.

Dr. Segredo attended The Florida State University, where she began her personal training career while pursuing her education. She graduated with Exercise Science and Business Management degrees and subsequently attended The University of South Florida where she graduated with her Doctor of Physical Therapy. She furthered her post-professional education with the completion of a neurologic residency program, which led to her becoming a Board Certified Neurologic Clinical Specialist.

She specializes in helping people who have sustained catastrophic injuries return back to living independent and fulfilling lives. She has worked across the healthcare continuum in settings from acute hospitals, inpatient rehabilitation centers, outpatient rehabilitation clinics, and home health. Dr. Segredo values education and paying it forward, and has played an integral part in mentoring doctoral students, residents, and fellow colleagues through her roles as a clinical mentor and didactic lecturer in residency programs, as well as in the development and teaching of continuing education courses.

Dr. Segredo has always had a strong passion for fitness and wellness, and takes pride in the fact that the gym is her favorite pastime. Having aging parents herself, she has energetically pursued a path to educate and encourage older adults to prioritize their health and wellness.

To ensure you get the most value and best experience out of your ageless fitness journey, click the link below to access your free supplemental material guide.

https://bit.ly/3x3FmbJ

CHAPTER 1

Introduction to Ageless Fitness

1.1 The Importance of Fitness in Older Adults

As we get older, prioritizing fitness becomes the key to living a fulfilled, high-quality life. Regular exercise promotes sound mental and emotional health, and goes beyond just making us stronger. In this book, we hope to provide a self-guide for older adults who wish to learn about the benefits of fitness and take the steps towards living a life which focuses on wellness in a safe, yet effective, manner in older adulthood.

Being physically active is the best way to deal with the challenges that come with getting older. Exercise is an important component of staying healthy, and helps slow down the process of your muscles and bones breaking down naturally as you age. Focusing on staying fit helps protect you from health problems that come with getting older, makes you more independent, and slows down the physical effects of getting older. Living an ageless fitness lifestyle is magical in many more ways than one--it keeps your mind sharp, keeps your emotions in check, and makes your life more enjoyable all around.

Fitness Guide for Older Adults

Whether you are an older adult starting out on your fitness journey, or an experienced and fit person going into your older adult life, you will benefit from a well-rounded plan that fits your needs at this point in your life. A complete exercise plan is important for maintaining and improving your health and overall quality of life. This routine should include different types of exercise, each serving their own purpose, with the end result being a comprehensive exercise plan which helps to promote and maintain an ageless fitness lifestyle.

Strength training is an integral component and type of exercise which should be included in an exercise program. Not only is it important to build muscle, but it also facilitates increased bone density, as well as helps provide the strength needed for daily tasks.

Cardiovascular exercises are an important part of any fitness plan, but they are especially important for older adults. Cardiovascular activities such as brisk walking, swimming, or cycling are great ways to keep the heart strong and working well without putting too much stress on the body. These exercises are good for the heart, and also improve lung capacity and endurance, making normal activities easier, such as walking up a flight of stairs. Cardio exercises can help you control your weight, blood sugar, and cholesterol levels, which is very important for avoiding or managing chronic conditions that become more common as we age.

Balance and stability training are essential components of fitness for older adults. Balance typically declines with age, increasing the risk of falls. It is important to integrate exercises that enhance balance and stability in your fitness program. Practices such as yoga and Tai Chi, along with simple activities like standing on one leg or walking heel-to-toe, significantly reduce the likelihood of falls and boost confidence in movement. These exercises are key to maintaining independence and safety with mobility. This form of exercise focuses on mimicking common daily movements such as bending down to tie shoes, reaching for items on high shelves, or briskly walking to catch a bus. The aim is to translate the strength, flexibility, and balance gained from regular exercise into practical, everyday abilities.

Including these activities in an exercise program can make a big difference in the quality of life for older people. The aim should be to tailor each person's exercise program so that it fits each person's needs and abilities. This customization ensures that the exercise plan is effective and fun, which encourages long-term commitment and consistency. The goal is for fitness to become a fun and healthy part of everyday life so that people can enjoy better health, more freedom, and a greater sense of well-being as they get older.

1.2 Benefits of Regular Exercise for Older Adults

A key component of health and wellbeing is regular exercise, especially as we age. It is an effective tool that does more than help prevent chronic diseases and maintain a healthy weight. Regular physical activity has many benefits for older individuals' physical, mental, and emotional well-being. This chapter emphasizes the many advantages of physical activity for the elderly population, stressing its potential as a preventative strategy as well as a means of improving quality of life.

Exercise is first and foremost crucial for preserving and enhancing bone density and muscle mass, both of which decline with age. An essential part of an older adult's exercise regimen is strength training, which halts this deterioration. Resistance training, such as lifting weights, strengthens bones in addition to building muscle. This increase in bone density is essential for lowering the risk of osteoporosis and fractures, which become increasingly common as people age. Furthermore, these strength training exercises directly improve daily function by reducing the difficulty of daily tasks such as carrying groceries.

Balance and stability are areas where regular exercise is also very beneficial. Targeted balance and stability exercises can considerably reduce falls, a key risk for seniors. Through the development of core strength, flexibility, and coordination, these exercises improve an individual's ability to move safely through daily life. Not only does better balance lower the chance of falling, but it also gives people more confidence when they move. Working on balance also helps to improve balance reactions, so that one is able to safely catch themselves or step to prevent a fall in a situation such as avoiding a moving crowd or quickly moving out of the way when a pet is nearing to try to jump up to say hi.

Walking, swimming, and cycling are fantastic ways to improve cardiovascular health. These heart-strengthening, low-impact cardio exercises are perfect for older adults because they do not cause overstraining. Frequent participation in these kinds of exercises strengthens the heart and lungs, increases energy, and enhances endurance—all of which support a more strenuous and active way of living.

Exercise can be a comforting salve for those suffering from arthritis or joint discomfort. Low-impact exercises like Tai Chi or water aerobics improve flexibility, reduce stiffness, and build stronger muscles around the joints. This strengthening offers pain and discomfort relief, and subsequently moving becomes less intimidating and more pleasurable.

Because it improves one's capacity to carry out daily tasks, functional training is particularly noteworthy. Functional training improves a person's ability to perform daily tasks with ease and independence by concentrating on specific movements such as bending, lifting, and reaching. This type of training is essential for preserving the ability to carry out daily tasks and maintaining a high quality of life.

Last but not least, regular exercise is a good way to address poor posture and back pain, which are also common as we age. Back discomfort can significantly decrease and posture can significantly improve with core strengthening and mobility-promoting workouts which focus on engaging the muscles of postural control, such as the upper back muscles, core, and glutes.

Older persons who regularly exercise can reap a wide range of life-changing benefits. Exercise plays a vital function in promoting physical fitness, preventing disease, improving mental health, and relieving joint pain. Older folks can experience enhanced strength, balance, flexibility, and general well-being by combining a range of activities catered to their individual needs. This will contribute to a healthier, more active, and overall satisfying life as they age.

1.3 Overcoming Barriers to Fitness in Older Age

Staying physically active is a crucial aspect of maintaining health and wellness in older age. However, several barriers can hinder regular exercise participation.

Knowledge and Guidance on Safe Exercise

It can be hard to find your way around the world of fitness, especially for older people who are more likely to get hurt and need to make sure they exercise safely. Lack of information or direction on how to exercise safely and successfully is a common barrier. This being an issue is part of the inspiration for creating this easy-access resource which provides comprehensive and clear instructions. The goal is to ensure you can safely and confidently perform different types of exercise which best fit your needs and preferences.

We all know that one size does not fit all when it comes to fitness, especially as we age. Allow *Ageless Fitness* to serve as a guide which provides flexibility, accommodations, and customizations that can be utilized by people with different levels of strength and mobility. Whether you have never worked out before, or are an experienced fitness guru, this self-guide will ensure that your workout plan fits your needs.

Managing Joint Pain and Discomfort

A lot of older people deal with joint pain and soreness daily, which makes it difficult for them to perform physical activities. Many people experience this pain because of disease processes like arthritis or simply the normal wear and tear of our joints and body that comes with getting older. Either way, this pain and discomfort can make it very hard to stay active. It is important to know that exercise can be a very useful tool for controlling and even getting rid of joint pain if done properly. There is a common misconception that exercise can make joint pain worse, but in fact, structured and well-designed exercise practices can help ease joint pain.

The importance of using the right form and skill in all exercises is a key part of this process. Form is important for more than just getting results--it is also important for safety, especially when it comes to protecting joints that are less flexible. In *Ageless Fitness* we incorporate workouts that are perfect for people with conditions such as arthritis because they focus on building strength and flexibility without putting too much stress on the joints. This resource emphasizes the importance of performing exercises in a proper way and maximizing their benefits without worsening any health problems.

Overcoming Physical Limitations

Physical restrictions can frequently be a major deterrent to regular exercise, especially for older persons. These restrictions might differ greatly from person to person and can result from long-term medical issues or just be a normal aspect of aging. They can range from diminished strength and endurance to impaired mobility and chronic pain. These difficulties may deter many people from exercising, which could result in a sedentary lifestyle that worsens existing health problems. It is crucial to realize, nevertheless, that these restrictions do not have to mean that an active life is over. Exercise can be a very effective technique for addressing these issues and enhancing overall health if done correctly.

This book provides a manual for overcoming these physical constraints through exercise. It yields methods for tailoring workout regimens to your unique requirements and capabilities. You will discover recommendations on which workouts to choose based on your current physical state and how to adapt them so they are safe and effective. The book offers a variety of adjustments to make every workout practical and efficient, such as modifying the range of motion, increasing the intensity, or utilizing assistive technology. You may reap the health advantages of physical activity while also honoring and adjusting to your body's demands by customizing your exercise regimen.

Addressing Mobility Challenges

Reduced mobility is one of the typical obstacles older persons confront while trying to maintain an active lifestyle. This obstacle may make it harder to utilize certain equipment or conventional training facilities, which could result in a decrease in physical activity. In *Ageless Fitness* we discuss how fitness is still achievable regardless of mobility capabilities. Our approach does not rely on a lot of equipment or access to a gym. We believe it's important to focus on a variety of workouts that are simple to complete at home. The simplicity and effectiveness of these workouts make them appropriate for a range of mobility levels and allow for easy integration into daily routines.

This book contains carefully selected workouts that are safe and effective for those with limited mobility. Their main goals are to improve balance, strength, and flexibility—all essential elements of total physical fitness. For example, chair exercises like leg lifts or sitting marches offer a low-impact approach to increase circulation and leg strength. Likewise, in order to strengthen the lower body and improving balance, one can perform standing exercises like side leg lifts and standing calf raises with the assistance of a chair or counter. Stretching and flexibility exercises can help to promote joint mobility and muscle relaxation.

Our method stresses how important it is to incorporate these motions into your everyday routine so that being active becomes a convenient and organic part of your day. This could be as easy as stretching your arms while watching TV, raising your calves while washing dishes, or sitting and gently twisting your body while performing deep breathing. This kind of integration not only increases accessibility to exercise but also aids in creating routines that are long-lasting. This strategy addresses the issue of decreased mobility by incorporating exercise into daily activities, making fitness a practical and pleasurable aspect of daily life for older adults.

Motivation and Mental Barriers

Staying motivated to engage in regular exercise can often be very difficult, with mental obstacles being a major contributing factor. These obstacles may include: a lack of interest in participating in physical activities, a fear of getting hurt, doubts about exercise's long-term benefits, or a lack of confidence on how to get started or even how to perform specific exercises. When it comes to committing to a fitness regimen, these mental obstacles can be just as restrictive as any physical barrier. *Ageless Fitness* provides purposeful strategies from evidence-based data and best practices that address these problems and emphasize the advantages of remaining active, particularly as one ages. Fitness in older adulthood involves more than just mindless performance of exercises. It involves changing one's attitude and view towards fitness in later life. This mental reframing provides a feeling of direction and purpose for one's fitness journey, serving as an effective motivator.

Financial Constraints

A common concern is that staying active through fitness programs or gym memberships can cost a lot of money. This idea that exercising is expensive can hinder and discourage people. It is important to dispel this myth and bring attention to the many low-cost or even free exercise choices that are perfect for older adults. Staying fit and healthy does not have to break the bank.

A lot of places offer free or low-cost fitness programs at local parks, community centers, or senior centers. These programs also offer you a chance to meet new people and socialize with your peers. Some insurance companies offer reduced, and sometimes free, gym membership options for retired or older adults. There are also free and useful online tools, such as exercise videos, instructional guides, and virtual classes, that can help people of all fitness levels and with different interests. These resources afford older people the opportunity to exercise in the comfort of their own homes, without having to pay for expensive gym memberships or equipment. Simple workouts that work well, such as walking, jogging, or strength and flexibility routines can be performed at home and do not require many, if any, special tools. This makes it easy to fit into your daily life.

1.4 Setting Realistic Fitness Goals for Older Adults

Setting realistic fitness goals is crucial to ensure that the goals are achievable, safe, and tailored to individual needs and abilities.

Here are some guidelines for setting realistic fitness goals:

- Consult with a Healthcare Professional: Before starting any fitness program, it is important to consult a healthcare provider. A healthcare professional can assess your health status and provide guidance on safe and suitable exercises.
- Consider Individual Health and Fitness Levels: Take your current health status, fitness level, and any existing medical conditions into account. Goals should be tailored to match each person's abilities and limitations.
- Focus on Functional Fitness: Emphasize goals that improve functional fitness such as flexibility, balance, and strength. These aspects are particularly important for maintaining independence and preventing falls.
- Set Specific, Measurable, Achievable, Relevant, and Time-Bound (SMART) Goals: Ensure that goals are SMART. For example, rather than a vague goal such as "get in shape," a SMART goal could be "walk for 30 minutes, 5 days/week, for the next 8 weeks."
- Gradual Progression: Start with realistic and attainable goals and then gradually progress over time. This approach helps prevent injuries and allows the body to adapt to new challenges.
- Regular Monitoring and Adjustments: Regularly monitor progress and be willing to adjust goals based on individual responses and changing circumstances. Flexibility is key to accommodating any physical changes or health considerations.

- Make it Enjoyable: Select activities that you enjoy. This increases motivation and adherence to the exercise routine.
- Include Social Elements: Consider activities that involve social interaction. This can enhance motivation and make the fitness journey more enjoyable.

The secret is to design an exercise plan that is safe, enduring, and tailored to each person's particular requirements and capabilities. As abilities or health conditions change over time, regular goal-setting and reevaluations may be required. Preserving your physical health depends upon setting reasonable fitness goals. The next chapters will discuss creating a customized fitness regimen that incorporates low-impact aerobics activities, strength training, joint pain treatment, functional training, posture correction, and back pain relief.

These recommendations can help you age gracefully, live better, and become more physically healthy overall.

CHAPTER 2

Fitness Guide for Older Adults

2.1 Assessing Fitness Levels in Older Adults

As we get older, taking care of our bodies and staying fit becomes more and more important. Regular exercise and other physical activities are important for more than just keeping in shape. They can also help improve the quality of life for older people and help prevent the chronic diseases that often come with getting older. It can help you not only live longer, but also enjoy a better quality of life.

Starting an exercise plan is not the same for everyone, especially as we get older. The body of each person has its own strengths and places that need more work. Because of this, you should always take the time to figure out what your baseline fitness levels are before starting an exercise routine. Assessing your fitness levels is an important step because it shows you exactly what parts of your health need work and can serve as a guide for selecting exercise for your fitness routine. Knowing your body's strengths and weaknesses is important for creating a workout plan that is safe and effective.

Before you start your fitness path it is crucial that you create a plan that fits your goals and physical abilities. Knowing where you stand prior to creating a customized routine is the first step to a purposeful and long-lasting fitness journey, whether your goal is to improve your cardiovascular health, get stronger, or become more flexible. This careful planning makes sure that you perform healthy activities without putting yourself at risk of injury, which sets you up for a happier and more active lifestyle as you age.

In this chapter, we will describe the reasoning, process, and inclusion of specific fitness assessments in your routine. Certain assessments and exercises will be generally described based on their applicability within each section for a foundational perspective, and will later be described in more detail within their respective chapters. You can also find detailed copies of these assessments and instructions on how to use them in the supplemental materials folder, under "Chapter 2." Click the link to access the supplemental material folder: https://bit.ly/3x3FmbJ.

Some key areas to consider when assessing your fitness levels as an older adult are:

Strength and Muscle Mass

Assessing your strength levels is a crucial step in creating a fitness program tailored for older adults. Focusing on maintaining muscle mass and preventing age-related muscle loss is essential. Here are some tests you can utilize to gauge your baseline strength:

Chair Stand Test

- Measures lower body strength and the ability to rise from a chair.
- Involves counting the number of times you can stand up and sit down in a specific time frame, typically 30 seconds or 1 minute.

Modified Push-Up Test

- Provides insight into upper body strength.
- Performed against a wall or on an incline, offering a less strenuous alternative to traditional push-ups.

Hand Grip Strength

- A simple yet effective measure of overall strength.
- Hand dynamometers are used for this test.
- Lower grip strength is often linked to functional decline in older adults.

Each of these tests helps in determining the right resistance and weight training exercises that suit your fitness level, enabling you to effectively maintain your strength as you age.

Balance and Stability

Assessing balance and stability is crucial to prevent falls and related injuries. Understanding your current balance abilities helps in choosing the right exercises to enhance coordination and stability. Here are key assessments to gauge balance and fall risk:

Berg Balance Scale

- A comprehensive tool comprising 14 different tasks.
- Includes activities like sitting to standing, standing unsupported, turning to look behind, and standing on one leg.
- Each task is scored based on performance.

Timed Up and Go (TUG) Test

- Measures the time taken to rise from a chair, walk 3 meters, turn around, walk back, and sit down.
- Assesses mobility, balance, functional movement, and speed.

Dynamic Gait Index (DGI)

- Evaluates the ability to modify gait during various tasks.

- Tasks include walking with head turns, navigating around obstacles, stepping over obstacles, and altering walking speed.

These assessments provide valuable insights into your balance and stability, guiding you to select exercises that improve these areas, thereby reducing your risk of falls and injuries.

Cardiovascular Health

Cardiovascular health is pivotal for older adults, and assessing it helps tailor the intensity and duration of aerobic exercises like walking, swimming, or cycling. Here are essential assessments to gauge cardiovascular fitness:

Six-Minute Walk Test

- Participants walk as fast as they can for 6 minutes.
- The distance covered is measured.
- This test estimates aerobic capacity and endurance.

Rate of Perceived Exertion (RPE) Scale

- The Borg RPE scale allows subjective rating of exertion level during exercise.
- Useful for monitoring exercise progress and adjusting intensity.

These assessments provide a clear picture of your cardiovascular health, enabling you to choose workouts that are effective yet safe, enhancing heart health and overall endurance.

Joint Pain Management

Joint pain management is crucial for older adults. Properly assessing joint health is key to tailoring exercises for pain relief and improved mobility. Here are essential assessments for joint integrity:

Range of Motion (ROM) Testing

- Measures the degree of movement in a joint.
- Performed actively (by the individual) or passively (by someone else).
- Assesses flexibility and identifies limitations or stiffness.

Pain Assessment

- Individuals report pain or discomfort experienced during specific movements.
- Includes noting the pain's location, intensity, and type.
- Provides vital information about joint health and areas needing attention.

These assessments guide the development of an exercise program focused on alleviating joint pain and enhancing joint mobility, crucial for maintaining an active lifestyle in older age.

Functional Training

Functional training is tailored to enhance the ability to perform daily activities. To determine your functional capabilities and identify areas for improvement, consider these assessments:

Functional Training Assessments

- Incorporate elements from other fitness assessments.
- Utilize the Chair Stand Test to evaluate lower body strength and functional mobility.
- Employ the Timed Up and Go (TUG) Test to assess mobility, balance, and speed of functional movements.
- Use specific tasks from the Berg Balance Scale for a comprehensive functional fitness assessment.
- Track changes and progress over time to gauge improvements in functional abilities.

These assessments help design a functional training program focused on daily life activities, ensuring older adults can continue to perform tasks like bending, lifting, and reaching with ease and efficiency.

Posture and Back Pain

Assessing posture and addressing back pain are crucial for maintaining health and well-being in older age. Proper posture assessment can help identify imbalances and guide corrective exercises. Here's how older adults can assess their posture:

Plumb Line Alignment

- Use a mirror or another person as a reference.
- Check alignment of key body parts: earlobe, shoulder, hip joint, knee joint, and ankle joint.
- Ensure the plumb line passes through these points when viewed from the side.

Digital Posture Analysis

- Utilize digital tools like posture analysis software or smartphone apps.
- These tools analyze posture using photographs or videos.

Postural Assessment Forms

- Employ structured checklists to evaluate posture.
- Document observations of various aspects of posture.

We will get into more detail regarding the breakdown and specifics of performing some of these assessments throughout this guide. These assessments can be performed with a professional, such as a physical therapist. However, you can also use them in a modified format, taking certain components from them and/or performing them on your own, in order to use them as a metric for self-monitoring throughout your fitness journey. Assessments done on a regular basis help create an exercise plan that fits each person's needs and goals. By checking in on your fitness levels on a regular basis, you can see how you are doing and make any necessary changes to your routine.

2.2 Designing a Safe and Effective Exercise Program

Regular exercise not only keeps you strong, but it also makes you feel better mentally and improves your quality of life as a whole. It is very important to make an exercise plan that is safe and effective and takes your specific needs and limits into account. We have already talked about how to set SMART goals and figure out your basic fitness levels. We can now focus on creating an exercise plan that is safe and effective. Outlined below are essential components to every person's exercise routine which can be modified based on each person's abilities and preferences.

Warm-Up

A full warm-up is an important first step in any exercise plan, but it is especially important for older people. It is important to slowly get the body ready for exercise, which can help avoid injuries and boost performance. A good warm-up should include a range of exercises that slowly raise the heart rate, open up the joints, and stretch the muscles in a dynamic way.

Light aerobic exercises are a great way to start because they get the blood moving. Walking quickly, riding a bike slowly, or even moving while standing still can all slowly raise the heart rate. After that, workouts for joint mobility help keep the joints loose and lubricated. Simple moves like arm circles, ankle rolls, and gentle twists can make joints more flexible and improve their range of motion. Adding dynamic stretches to the end of the warm-up gets the muscles ready for the upcoming exercises.

These are active moves that stretch muscles without holding them in the end position. This way of warming up ensures the body is ready, which lowers the risk of strain or injury and sets the stage for a more effective and enjoyable workout.

Cardiovascular Exercise

Cardiovascular exercises should be a regular part of your weekly practice to keep your heart healthy, especially as you get older. Performing aerobic exercises regularly can help protect against heart disease and improve your health in general. It is important for older people to do workouts that are both good for them and easy on their bodies.

Brisk walking, cycling, swimming, and low-impact aerobics are all great cardiovascular sports for adults. They are easy on the joints and can be enjoyable, which makes them great for staying fit as you get older. The level of intensity for these exercises should depend on the person, but a low to moderate level of intensity is ideal. A good rule of thumb is to keep your heart rate between 50 and 70% of its highest (Max HR) for 30 minutes, 4-5 times a week at the very least. The easy way to find your Max HR is to take 220 and subtract your age. It is best to build up to this level of energy slowly, starting with the level of fitness you already have and steadily getting progressing. This method makes sure that there is a safe and effective way to improve cardiovascular health that takes into account how your body changes as you age.

Balance and Stability

Adding balance and stability exercises to your workout routine is very important, especially if you want to lower your risk of falling, which is a common worry for older people. Start by focusing on the areas where your first assessments of balance showed there was room for change. It is important to do these routines at least three times a week. During each lesson, you should do each exercise several times. As your fitness and confidence improve, you should gradually increase the number of times you do each exercise and the difficulty of these exercises. A standard method for progressing balance exercises is to gradually decrease the assistance from your arms while performing the exercise, and to progress from a stable surface to a more compliant, or dynamic, surface, when performing the exercise.

Flexibility Training

As you get older, it is especially important to keep your joints mobile and less stiff by doing flexibility exercises. At the end of every workout, make it a habit to do static stretching movements for the main muscle groups. This practice helps to lengthen muscles, make them more flexible, and lower the risk of soreness and pain after exercise.

Progression

Progression in your exercise routine is key to achieving continuous improvement and avoiding plateaus. As you notice advancements in your fitness levels, it's important to gradually increase various aspects of your workout regimen.

This means methodically enhancing the frequency of your workouts, extending their duration, stepping up the intensity, and introducing more challenging exercises.

This approach ensures that your body is consistently being challenged, which is crucial for ongoing physical development. As you progress, you'll find yourself able to handle more demanding workouts, and this escalation should be tailored to your individual improvements. Remember, the goal is to steadily push your limits while remaining attentive to your body's responses, ensuring a balanced and effective fitness journey.

Monitoring and Adaptation

It is important to keep an eye on and change your exercise plan on a regular basis. Performing regular reassessments that are in line with your initial baseline surveys can help you see how you are doing and help you make any necessary changes. These check-ins let you change your exercise plan based on things like your changing pain levels, your progress, your personal schedule, your exercise preferences, and your general performance.

By making changes to your routine based on these new findings, you can keep your workout safe, effective, and fun. Making these changes is very important, whether it is changing the speed, the length, or the activities to fit your changing fitness levels or interests. Keeping up with these changes helps you keep your exercise plan flexible and adaptable, so it can fit your unique path to better health and well-being.

Hydration and Recovery

Ensuring adequate hydration and prioritizing sufficient rest and recovery are fundamental for a successful fitness regimen, especially for older adults. It's vital to understand the importance of drinking enough water before, during, and after exercise to maintain optimal body function and performance. Proper hydration aids in muscle recovery, joint lubrication, and overall improvement of our bodies physiological processes.

Additionally, allowing adequate time for rest and recovery is crucial in any exercise program. This not only helps in preventing overuse injuries but also ensures that the body has time to repair and strengthen itself. It's important for older adults to be well-informed about the benefits of exercise, nutritional needs, correct execution of exercises, and the overall safety and sustainability of their fitness routines, which includes recovery-based strategies and principles.

Social Engagement

Including social aspects in your fitness routine can make you much more motivated to stick to a daily exercise schedule. Working out with other people your age or with friends not only makes the activities more fun, but it also gives them a sense of community and support. Joining a walking club, taking group classes, or even just working out with other people can really help you stick with your exercise plan.

When making an exercise plan for older people that is safe and successful, it is important to make sure that it fits their needs and limitations. Start with easy workouts and slowly build up the volume as your body gets used to them. Pay close attention to how your body feels before, during, and after workouts. Living a busy and healthy life as an older person can have many benefits, such as better physical and mental health and more social connections.

2.3 Incorporating Strength Training for Older Adults

Incorporating strength training into your fitness routine as you get older is not just about exterior physical appearance or "looking big and fit." It is also about staying independent and making your life better in general. Your muscles naturally get weaker with age, which makes you more likely to hurt yourself or fall. By strength training regularly, you can actively fight this decline and make sure you can continue to live your life to the fullest.

Strength training is very important for joint health. Building up the muscles around your joints gives them support and stability and eases the stress on the joints themselves. This helps combat areas that may be painful we age, like the hips or knees. Focusing on specific exercises can help you build the muscle support you need to ease pain in these places.

Aside from facilitating independence and decreased joint pain, strength training also has a significant impact on bone density maintenance. Maintaining bone density is vital in the prevention and slowing down of osteoporosis, a common issue which occurs with age. Increased muscle mass also results in improved stability and balance, which lowers the chance of falls, which are a major source of injuries among the elderly. Strength training can also increase one's metabolic rate, which helps control blood sugar levels and aids in weight management. This is especially advantageous for people who are managing illnesses such as type 2 diabetes.

When it comes to suggested exercise, the emphasis should be on joint-friendly, low-impact activities that work the main muscle groups. Resistance band exercises, light free-weight lifts, leg presses, and seated rowing are all great options. These can be done at home with little equipment or with gym equipment. It is important to begin with smaller weights and build resistance gradually as your strength increases. This steady progression reduces the chance of injury while also promoting muscle growth. Older folks should be aware of their body's signals and prioritize their safety. Stopping any exercise that hurts more than your average muscular tiredness is the best course of action. Assuring that exercises are performed correctly and safely, with the proper form, is imperative for successful execution of a strength training program.

2.4 Utilizing Balance and Stability Exercises for Seniors

It is important to make balance and steadiness a priority in your workouts. You can avoid falls and injuries by doing these kinds of workouts, but they also make your life better in other important ways. Let us talk about how doing balance and stability exercises can help you, especially if you are older, and then look at some good exercises.

Balance and stability routines are very important if you want to stay independent and feel more confident in the things you do every day. Doing these exercises daily will make your muscles stronger, your coordination better, and your joints more flexible. All of these things will make you less likely to fall. Fall prevention is extremely important to avoid breaking a bone or other serious injuries. When you work on your balance and stability, you can keep up a busier, fast-paced lifestyle without having to worry about safety with your mobility.

The single-leg stand is an example of a good exercise to add to your practice. To begin, hold on to a strong chair or counter for balance. Take one leg off the ground and hold it there for 10 to 15 seconds. Then move on to the other leg. As you get stronger, try balancing without hanging on to anything for an extra challenge.

The heel-toe walk is another good practice. Place one foot in front of the other on the floor in a straight line, and walk along the line. The heel-toe movement improves your coordination and builds power in your core and legs.

You can also get better balance and stability by doing yoga and tai chi. These gentle, low-impact workouts are all about being aware of your body and moving in a controlled way. You can make these habits a part of your daily life by taking a class in person or following online lessons.

By setting aside time for stability and balance routines, you are taking the first step toward a healthier, more active life. Perform these movements to get stronger and more flexible, and enjoy the extra confidence and freedom they give you in your daily life as they improve your balance.

2.5 Implementing Low-Impact Cardio Workouts for Seniors

Regular exercise keeps bones and muscles strong, keeps your heart healthy, and helps you control your weight. Older people who have joint pain, arthritis, or other physical injuries or health issues may not be able to perform high-impact exercise workouts. This is why low-impact exercise workouts are preferred.

Although they are easier on the joints, low-impact cardio workouts are still good for the heart. They also build stamina, and burn calories while preventing overall pain and strain on your body. There are several low-impact cardio workouts designed for older adults that can help achieve cardiovascular health and fitness.

Walking is an example of a great low-impact workout. You can change it to fit your exercise level and it is easy on your joints. Regular walking, whether it is a slow stroll through the park, or a fast stroll through the neighborhood, is good for your heart, makes your legs stronger, and helps you stay at a healthy weight.

Swimming and water exercises are also great low-impact choices. Because the water is buoyant, it lessens the pressure on the joints, making these exercises great for people with arthritis or joint pain. Working out in the water makes you more flexible, stronger, and builds endurance.

Biking, even stationary biking, is a low-impact cardio workout that builds energy, strengthens leg muscles, and improves balance. Cycling outside allows you to get fresh air, which can make the exercise more fun and therapeutic. Stationary bikes are a safe and handy option for people who would rather, or need to, stay inside. Biking is a good cardio workout option and does not put too much stress on your joints.

No matter what age you are, you can live a fit and active life if you design the right workout plan. So put on your walking shoes, jump in the pool, or ride your bike, and enjoy the health benefits of low-impact exercise workouts tailored around the needs of older people. It is both good for your mind and your body.

2.6 Managing Joint Pain through Exercise for Seniors

Joint discomfort can worsen with age and have a major influence on your daily activities and general health. There is hope and a solution for this, though--you can control, and even lessen, your discomfort with the correct exercise regimen.

Controlling your joint pain is an essential component of any workout. Low-impact exercises, range-of-motion exercises, and gentle stretching are good ways to improve joint mobility and reduce inflammation.

One important way to deal with joint pain is to warm up before each work out and stretch properly after each workout. Warm-up activities get the body ready for more active movements by slowly getting circulation going in preparation for more difficult and intense movements. This occurs by increasing blood flow to the muscles and joints, which makes them less stiff and painful. Arm circles, shoulder shrugs, and gentle walking in place are all simple exercises that can serve as a warm-up. Also, stretching is very important because it helps maintain and increase flexibility, which is imperative for joint health. When you stretch, you should be gentle and never move a joint past its natural range of motion. You should focus on all of your major joints, like your shoulders, wrists, hips, knees, and ankles.

Older adults can manage joint pain by performing exercises such as water aerobics, walking, or stationary riding, all of which are low-impact exercises. These exercises are considered physical exercise, which is good for your health in general, without putting too much stress on your joints. Working on strength training is also important because bigger muscles support and protect the joints. But when you work out, it is important to use light weights and move slowly and carefully. Using resistance bands is a good way to perform strength training because they are easy on the joints while allowing you to change the amount of resistance.

Adding these movements to your daily or weekly routine can make your joints much more flexible, strong, and mobile overall. It is important to pay close attention to your body and avoid performing movements that cause pain. By putting joint health first and doing the right exercises, seniors can take charge of their joint pain and live a more comfortable, but busy, life.

By controlling joint discomfort with a thorough exercise regimen, you may preserve and improve your joint health, mobility, and overall quality of life. You can successfully manage joint discomfort and lead an active, healthy lifestyle by combining strength training, balance and stability exercises, low-impact aerobic workouts, functional training, and an emphasizing correct posture and form.

2.7 Enhancing Functional Training for Daily Activities in Older Age

It becomes increasingly important to be able to carry out our daily duties efficiently and independently as we get older. Incorporating functional training is essential because it is task-specific training which mirrors our daily responsibilities and activities. The main goals of this kind of training are to increase your strength, flexibility, balance, and coordination in order to be able to safely and effectively remain independent with all of your daily lifestyle tasks.

The goal of functional training is to simulate common actions like bending, reaching, lifting, and walking during your exercise routine. As an older adult, this approach is especially helpful since it increases your physical functional abilities, improves your posture and balance, and lowers your risk of injury and falls.

Functional training exercises typically consist of compound movement exercises, which work out a lot of muscle groups at once, focusing on coordination, balance, and power. For example, the squat-to-chair and step-up movements are like sitting down and getting up from a chair or climbing stairs. These workouts not only make your legs and lower back stronger, but they also make you more stable and improve your balance, all while simulating common everyday movements and activities. Similarly, arm raises and light weightlifting can help you mimic actions like reaching overhead, which is useful for tasks like hanging clothes or organizing cabinets.

Functional training also includes moves that make you more flexible and increase your range of motion, which is important for jobs that require you to bend and twist. Some great exercises for keeping your spine and hips open are the seated twist and the standing hip hinges. Performing these exercises which maintain multi-joint flexibility makes it less likely that you will hurt yourself during everyday tasks. Balance movements like walking heel-toe or standing on one leg can also be incorporated into functional training and will help keep older people from falling, which can be a big fear or worry in older age.

To get the most out of functional training and lower your risk of injury, it is important to pay attention to form and controlled actions. You should start with a low level of light weight and slowly increase it as your strength and confidence grow. By adding functional training to your normal exercise routine, everyday tasks become easier to perform, which can help you live a more independent and enjoyable life.

2.8 Improving Posture and Relieving Back Pain in Elderly Individuals

As people age, problems like bad posture and back pain often have a big impact on their quality of life. Focused exercises and good habits can relieve back pain and improve posture.

To improve your posture, you need to work on developing your core muscles. These include the muscles in your stomach, back, and pelvic floor. Movements like wall sits, bridge poses, and pelvic tilts can be very helpful and are examples of core strengthening exercises. The core muscles play a large role in keeping your spine straight and supporting it. Performing strength training exercises that target these core muscles will improve your posture, and in turn, relieve back pain.

Workouts and stretches that focus on the muscles in your back can help ease back pain. Workouts that focus on strengthening your lower back muscles such as performing weighted back extension, stretches for your hamstrings and hip flexors, and gentle spinal twists all facilitate increased strength and flexibility and relieve stress in the back muscles.

Incorporating a regular stretching routine can help with both improving your posture and also easing back pain. When you stretch, you open up tight muscles and help combat muscle imbalances, which are often to blame for bad posture and back pain. It can help a lot to incorporate some light stretches for your neck, shoulders, back, and legs. For example, the sitting spinal twist and the cat-cow stretch can help make your spine more flexible.

Another important part of this methodology is incorporating techniques for keeping all of your major muscles and joints in the correct alignment. Good posture is something that seniors can work on every day, whether they are sitting, standing, or walking. Some tips that can really help are sitting with your feet flat on the ground, using lumbar support for your lower back, making sure your computer screen is at eye level, and not slouching. If you keep up with these habits, your posture will get better over time.

Remember that being consistent is very important if you want to improve your posture and alleviate back pain. Making these exercises and techniques a daily part of your life will make sure that these effects last and improve over time.

Ultimately, getting better posture and easing back pain takes a multifaceted approach that includes working on your core strength, flexibility, back muscles, overall body alignment, balance, and functional training. In your later years, you can improve your overall health, get better posture, and lessen back pain by using these tips and adding them to your everyday fitness routine.

CHAPTER 3

Strength Training for Older Adults

3.1 The Benefits of Strength Training in Older Age

Strength training is a vital component of fitness at any age, and can provide significant benefits for older adults when performed appropriately. Strength training becomes more crucial as we age to preserve bone density, muscular mass, and general physical functional ability. We have introduced the importance and the benefits to strength training as it relates to a lifestyle of ageless fitness in the first two chapters of this book. Now we will delve into more details and specifics of the benefits of strength training in older adulthood, and then move on to provide practical and detailed strategies that you may incorporate into your fitness routine as an older adult seeking to live an ageless fitness lifestyle.

STRENGTH TRAINING FOR OLDER ADULTS

The maintenance of muscle mass is one of the main advantages of strength training as you become older. Muscle loss associated with aging inevitably results in weakness, decreased mobility, and an increased risk of falls. By encouraging the building of new muscle fibers, resistance training counteracts this loss of muscle. This leads to better physical performance as well as increased strength.

Strength training is also essential for preserving bone density. For older folks, osteoporosis—a disorder characterized by weakening bones—is a serious worry. Weight-bearing activities that strengthen bones, such as lunges and squats, lower the risk of fractures. This preservation of bone density through the performance of closed chain weight bearing activities is greatly enhanced by the consistent performance of strength training.

Strength exercise can be quite helpful for senior citizens who are experiencing joint pain. It relieves joint stress and pain by strengthening the muscles around joints and stabilizing them. This can help reduce the risk of injury and improve joint function.

Building muscle through strength training can boost metabolism, making it easier for older adults to manage weight and body composition. Incorporating strength training into your fitness routine can also assist with combating chronic disease. Regular strength training has been associated with better management of chronic conditions such as arthritis, diabetes, and heart disease.

As mentioned in the first two chapters of this book, strength training improves balance and coordination, reducing the risk of falls, which is a common concern among older adults. Increased strength can enhance an individual's ability to perform daily activities, promoting independence and a higher quality of life.

Strength also has a positive effect on mental health, which should not go unnoticed. It can reduce symptoms of depression and anxiety and promote cognitive function. It can also contribute to better sleep patterns and overall sleep quality. Participating in group strength training classes or exercising with a partner can provide social interaction, reducing feelings of isolation and promoting a sense of community.

Strength training is an essential component of an active, healthy lifestyle for older adults. Its benefits include preservation of muscle mass, preservation of bone density, improvement of joint pain, improvement of metabolic and multi-system health, improvement in balance and stability, and mental health benefits. Strength training is a vital component of fitness regimens that older persons can incorporate to enhance their physical health and quality of life. This Chapter will provide information and guidance regarding equipment, parameters, and specific exercises. For additional information, including pictures of equipment discussed in this chapter and videos demonstrating each exercise, visit the "Chapter 3" folder in your supplemental material resource at https://bit.ly/3x3FmbJ.

3.2 Selecting Appropriate Resistance and Equipment

As you get older, it is important to keep up with and build upon a regular exercise routine. Selecting the right resistance and gear is a very important component of safety and efficiency of a strength training workout.

If you are an older adult, you should start strength training with lighter weights and higher reps. This method gradually increases strength and stamina, which lowers the risk of injury and ensures that your muscles are worked out properly without putting too much stress on your joints. Starting with lighter weight or resistance also allows the individual to focus on proper form and technique without risking injury. The appropriate weight or resistance level will vary per individual, and largely depends on their baseline fitness level. A good go-to self-guide for an older adult when choosing a resistance level is to choose a resistance level that allows for 10-15 repetitions with good form. If the weight is so light that the individual can easily perform more than 15 repetitions, consider increasing the resistance slightly. If they struggle to complete 10 repetitions with proper form, the weight may be too heavy. Incrementally increase or decrease the resistance based on these performance guidelines, then reassess, and adjust accordingly. This strategy of selecting weight and resistance levels will allow for a safe and effective gradual build in strength and muscle tone.

There are several suitable exercise equipment options that will facilitate a safe, yet productive, workout experience for building strength. Resistance bands are versatile and provide resistance for strength training without the need for heavy weights. Light dumbbells or free weights are also an option, as long as they are comfortable to hold and not so heavy that they compromise form. Weight tools with settings that allow you to change the resistance level are also a viable option. Stability balls can be used for core exercises and balance training. Consider exercises that can be performed using a sturdy chair. This provides support for those with balance issues and allows for seated workouts. Progressive resistance training selectorized machines with back support and fixed seats are an excellent option for isolating and strengthening major muscle groups in a safe and stable fashion. Using machines with easy-to-use controls and pictures, larger buttons, and added stability features such as handles, are some other important criteria to consider when selecting and using strength training equipment.

Aside from choosing the appropriate resistance (intensity) and equipment (mode), it is imperative to carefully consider customizing other components of your strength training routine such as frequency and duration. Starting at a frequency of 2-3 days per week is sufficient to establish a routine and start to see and feel the benefits of strength training. As fitness levels increase, increase frequency to 4, then 5, days/week to continue to see benefits and to obtain a training effect. A good indicator for increasing frequency is when you've been at the same frequency for about 3-4 weeks, you stop feeling muscle soreness after workouts, and you perceive the exercise to feel "easy" or "easy to moderate." An increase in frequency should always feel comfortable and should not cause pain or debilitating stiffness. Minor muscle soreness or fatigue are expected due to the change in activity. Remember to always reassess how you feel after any change in your workout routine, and make necessary adjustments.

Duration of strength training workouts should be based on how many muscle groups you are training that day and how many sets and repetitions are being performed of each exercise. A guideline that is safe and effective to follow is training all major upper body muscles one day of the week and all major lower body muscles another day, performing 2 strengthening exercises per muscle group, 3 sets of 10-15 repetitions for each exercise. This would mean strength training 2 days per week as a starting point, and progressively increasing as mentioned above. It is safe, and in fact, recommended, to perform other types of exercises on the same day, such as cardiovascular, balance, or postural training exercises, which would increase the overall duration of your workout.

Remember to keep it organized and structured, but also fun! Write out a plan of how many days per week, and how much time each day, you want to spend working out, and then fill in the blanks with a combination of the different types of workouts you want to include in your week based on the information you've been given thus far and your ageless fitness goals. Every 3-4 months—reassess and slightly change it up. It keeps the body on its toes and keeps the mind excited!

Recovery is an important component of an ageless fitness lifestyle. Stretching, modalities such as heat and/or ice, compression, massage, and postural work are integral components of recovery.

Equipment that may be helpful for recovery can include stretch bands/loops, foam rolls, massage guns, ice packs, heating pads, and compression sleeves.

3.3 Upper Body Strength Exercises

Upper body strengthening exercises should be performed for all major muscle groups as part of an effective strength training routine. Upper body strength affects many daily tasks and your ability to move freely during many functional tasks that you may not even recognize or consciously think about. Some examples are: opening jars, carrying groceries, reaching in cabinets, washing your hair, vacuuming, etc. As we age, maintaining strength is not just about staying fit--it is also about staying independent and making it easier to do everyday activities. Strength training for your upper body keeps your muscles in your arms, shoulders, chest, and back strong and capable of keeping up with your active lifestyle.

Here are some safe and effective upper body strengthening exercises specifically tailored for older adults:

Bicep Curls

- Use light dumbbells or resistance bands. Stand or sit with arms at your sides, palms facing forward. Slowly lift the weights toward your shoulders, then lower them back down.

Tricep Dips

- Use a sturdy chair. Sit on the edge with hands gripping the front of the chair. Slide your bottom off of the chair, lower yourself toward the floor, then push back up.

Overhead Press

- Sit or stand with light dumbbells. Lift the weights from shoulder height to overhead, extending your arms fully. Lower them back down with control.

Lateral Raises

- Hold light weight in each hand, arms at your sides. Lift your arms out to the sides until they are parallel to the ground, then lower them back down.

Shoulder Blade Squeezes

- Sit or stand with arms at your sides. Squeeze your shoulder blades together, hold for a moment, then release. This helps improve posture.

Wall Push-Ups

- Stand facing a wall, arms extended at chest height. Perform push-ups against the wall, keeping your body in a straight line.

Seated Rows

- Use resistance bands or cable machines. Sit with a straight back, and pull the handles toward you, squeezing your shoulder blades together.

Chest Press

- Lie on your back on a bench or the floor with light dumbbells in your hands and your elbows bent to 90 degrees. Press the weights up from the chest level, then lower them back down.

Wrist Curls

- Sit with your forearms resting on your thighs, holding a light weight in each hand. Curl the wrists up and down to work the forearm muscles.

Forearm Pronation and Supination

- Hold a light weight in each hand with palms facing up, elbows at your side and bent to 90 degrees. Rotate your forearms, turning the palms down and then back up.

Arm Circles

- Stand with arms extended to the sides. Make small circles with your arms, gradually increasing the size. Reverse the direction.

These exercises target all of the major muscle groups in the upper body. They are specifically geared towards older adults because the weight can be modified and self-selected, and the positioning for performing them facilitates good posture, especially because some of them can be performed while sitting down in a chair with back support. Once you begin to include these workouts in your regimen, you will see how they improve both your life and your fitness.

3.4 Lower Body Strength Exercises

Lower body strengthening is crucial to include in a well-rounded fitness routine for an older adult. Strengthening your lower body has many health benefits, such as increasing muscle mass in your lower extremity, improving overall balance and stability, improving coordination and agility, maintaining flexibility and range of motion, and in turn, being able to perform daily activities with much more ease and speed. Concentrating on your buttocks, hips, and legs strengthens your entire lower body.

Outlined below are a series of lower body strength training exercises that will help you meet your strength training goals and should be included in your strength training routine:

Bodyweight Squats

- Stand with feet hip-width apart. Lower your body as if sitting back into a chair, keeping your knees over your ankles. Stand back up.

Lunges

- Take a step forward with one foot and lower your body until both knees are bent at a 90-degree angle. Return to the starting position and repeat with the other leg.

Step-Ups

- Use a stable platform or step. Step up with one foot, bringing the other foot up beside it. Step back down and repeat on the other side.

Leg Press

- Use a leg press machine at the gym or a resistance band. Press your feet forward against the resistance, then return to the starting position. If using a resistance band, hold the ends of the band in your hands and wrap the middle part of the band around the bottom of your feet, at the level of the balls of your feet.

Calf Raises

- Stand on a flat surface, rise up onto your toes, and then lower your heels back down. You can do this exercise while holding onto a sturdy surface for balance.

Seated Leg Lifts

- Sit in a chair with your back straight. Lift one leg straight out in front of you and hold for 1-3 seconds. Lower it back down and repeat with the other leg.

Wall Sit

- Stand with your back flat against a wall and lower your body into a seated position, as if sitting in an imaginary chair. Hold for as long as comfortable. Incrementally add time as able/tolerated.

Hip Abduction/Adduction

- Use resistance bands, a pillow/ball, or a selectorized training machine. Move your legs outward (abduction) and inward (adduction) against resistance while keeping the other leg stable.

Side Leg Raises

- While standing or lying on your side, lift one leg sideways, then lower it back down. Repeat on the other side.

Hamstring Curls

- Use resistance bands or a machine. In standing or lying on your stomach, curl your heels toward your buttocks, engaging the hamstrings. If using resistance bands, tie the bands to a fixed, stable object at the same height, or slightly below, the level of your legs. The further you are from the band, the more tension/resistance you will feel. Wrap the middle part of the band around your ankles, and curl your heels as mentioned above.

These exercises target all of the major muscle groups in the lower body. They can be performed at home with a self-selected weight, or even bodyweight, or at a gym with specific machines which are used to perform these movements, as mentioned above. You will experience noticeable increases in joint health, muscle mass, and stability if you dedicate yourself to these strengthening workouts.

3.5 Core and Abdominal Strength Exercises

As you age, it becomes increasingly important to have a strong and stable core. A strong core is essential for many activities you do every day and for your general health. It plays a large role in helping you keep your balance, which is especially important to avoid falls. A strong core can also help with alleviating back pain, which is a problem that can really put a damper on the quality of life for many adults. By working on building your core, you can ease pain and make it easier to participate in everyday tasks. A solid core is also an integral part in maintaining straight and upright posture. It is the foundation for stability in your body, and will help prevent overuse and misuse of other muscles during everyday tasks if you strengthen it and learn how to engage it when performing activities.

Prioritizing core strength as you get older is an investment in your health and your future. It protects against injuries, especially those that involve balance and back problems, increases range of motion in multiple planes and directions, and makes you more stable overall. Building core strength is not just about having a six pack--it is about taking care of an important part of your body that helps and improves everything you do. You can improve your health and have a better quality of life in your older years by keeping your core strong and steady.

Below is a straightforward and easily self-performed guide to core and abdominal strength training exercises designed for older adults:

Plank

- Start on your hands and knees, then straighten your legs behind you, keeping your body in a straight line. Hold for as long as comfortable, engaging the core. To modify, perform on your knees or against a wall.

Bird-Dog

- Start on your hands and knees. Lift and extend one arm and the opposite leg, then switch sides. Keep your back flat and engage your core. To modify, stay on your knees and extend one arm, working toward lifting the opposite leg while you keep the arm extended.

Seated Torso Twist

- Sit tall in a chair with feet flat on the floor. Twist your torso to one side, hold for a moment, and then twist to the other side.

Leg Raises

- Lie on your back with legs straight. Lift one leg a few inches off the ground, then lower it back down. Switch legs and repeat. To modify, sit on the edge of a chair and lift your knees towards your chest, engaging your core.

Pelvic Tilts

- Lie on your back with your knees bent and your feet flat on the floor. Tighten your abdominal muscles and press your lower back into the floor, then release.

Superman

- Lie on your stomach with arms extended in front of you. Lift your arms, chest, and legs off the ground, engaging your back and core muscles.

Crunches

- Lie on your back with knees bent, hands behind your head. Lift your head and shoulders, focusing on your abs.

To maintain an ageless fitness lifestyle, you need to stay committed to your fitness path. As part of this commitment, you should work out regularly, eat well, and make decisions that will benefit your health and well-being in the long run. It is important to remember that getting fit is a marathon, not a sprint. It means making choices that are consistent and long-lasting that are good for your health and wellness as a whole. Maintaining a strong and healthy core will greatly improve your quality of life if you work at it consistently.

3.6 Designing a Well-Rounded Strength Training Routine

Regardless of age, strength training is an important part of any exercise plan. It is especially important for older people to maintain their muscle strength, as it is beneficial for their health and helps them stay independent. Most of us typically lose muscle strength as we get older, making strength training in late adulthood even more important. As we've discussed throughout this chapter, a well-planned strength training program not only helps you maintain and build your muscle mass, but it also helps with many other parts of your health and daily life.

A strength training program can greatly improve your functional skills. This makes it easier to handle daily jobs and activities that may have become harder with age and deconditioning. Strength training leads to a more active and independent way of life. Strength training is also a great way to deal with joint pain, which is common as we age. By making the muscles around the joints stronger, these workouts can ease pain and improve mobility by decreasing stress, wear, and tear on the joints, making moving around easier and less painful. A well-rounded strength exercise program is also very important for improving stability and balance. This is especially important for older people because it lowers their risk of falling, which is a big problem for people in this age group. By doing activities that make your muscles stronger you can improve your balance and stability, which can help you move more safely and with more confidence. Adding strength training to your fitness routine as you get older is not just a way to stay fit, it is also a way to improve your quality of life by maintaining your freedom, decreasing your pain, and making you more stable overall.

Let's break down how to craft an effective strength training plan:

Tailor to Your Needs

- Consult Professionals: Before starting, consult with a healthcare professional or a certified fitness trainer specializing in older adults.
- Utilize appropriate resources: Use safe and informative self-guided material to lead you and keep you organized and accountable (i.e.: *Ageless Fitness* book, online videos

and tutorials from trusted sources, friends or family who are experienced).
- Personalize Your Routine: Focus on your specific fitness goals and any health limitations you might have.

Target Major Muscle Groups

- Key Exercises: Include squats, lunges, push-ups, and planks to build strength in your legs, arms, back, and core.
- Add Resistance: Use tools like resistance bands or light dumbbells to challenge your muscles appropriately.

Create a Schedule

- Weekly Split/Schedule: Organize a weekly schedule where you are splitting up the muscles you are training into groups (i.e.: upper body and lower body) and deciding how many days per week you are training each group. Plan so that you give each group sufficient rest before strength training that group again. Increase frequency as you reassess and progress, and then adjust/change your schedule accordingly. Incorporate your other forms of exercise in combination with or around the days you strength train. Staying structured and organized creates positive habits and consistency, leading to a lifestyle change.

Warm-Up

- Start with 5-10 minutes of light aerobic or any form of dynamic activity, such as brisk walking, cycling, or mobility/agility training, to increase blood flow to the muscles in preparation for strengthening. This helps prevents injury and stiffness.

Cool Down

- Finish with 5-10 minutes of light aerobic activity, followed by static stretching. This helps prevent muscle stiffness and promotes flexibility.

Incorporate Other Types of Exercise

- We go through all of the different types of exercises that are specifically important for the older adult population in *Ageless Fitness*. It is essential to combine these various modes of exercise and not just focus on one of them in order to create a healthy and well-rounded fitness experience.
- Other types of exercises that should be incorporated with your strength training routine are: cardiovascular training, balance and stability exercises, functional training, postural training, and stretching/flexibility training.
- These exercises can be incorporated with strength training in the same day to ensure a comprehensive workout routine. There are various options for organizing a complete workout, and how you organize each day

largely depends on your time in each specific day and your schedule. An example of a full workout for one day is: 5 minute warm up, 30 minute upper body strength training, 30 minute cardiovascular training, 5 minute cool down, stretching. Another example is: 10 minute warm up, 30 minute lower body strength training, 5 minute cool down, 15 minute balance training exercises, 15 minute postural exercises, stretching. A third example is: 5 minute warm up, 15 minute brisk walk, 15 minute core strength training, 15 minute cycling, 10 minute balance and stability training, 10 minute functional training movements, 5 minute cool down, stretching. Depending on your baseline fitness level, you can always start at a comfortable point and incrementally build up to these examples.

Progression

- Gradually reassess progress and increase intensity, frequency, and duration as the individual becomes more fit. Ensure progression is gradual to prevent injury or overexertion. Changes may also need to occur (progress or scale back) as health needs or schedules change/fluctuate.

Recovery

- Rest and recovery are just as important as strength training when living an all-around ageless fitness lifestyle. Stretching, massage, foam rolling, postural training, proper nutrition, sleep, and mindfulness are all integral components of recovery which lead to recharging and therefore ultimately enhanced performance during strength training workouts.

As an older adult living an ageless fitness lifestyle, there are a wide range of components and guidelines to follow in order to maximize your strength training routine. This practice should focus on working out the body's main muscle groups, which is very important for keeping the body strong and functional as a whole. Strength training inadvertently facilitates increased balance, posture, flexibility, endurance, independence with functional tasks, and joint pain management due to its benefits. However, it is still essential to isolate and focus on these other components of exercise in addition to strength training in order to reap the benefits of a comprehensive ageless fitness lifestyle.

You can make a big difference in your fitness level and overall health by sticking to a regular and varied strength training routine. This consistent effort will not only help you stay independent, but it will also improve your quality of life, making it easier and less painful for you to perform daily tasks and stay active in both business and leisure activities.

CHAPTER 4

Balance and Stability Exercises

4.1 The Importance of Balance and Stability in Older Age

A training regimen that emphasizes stability and balance is essential as you age. Maintaining your quality of life while lowering the potential of injury from falls is possible with good balance and stability. In this chapter, we will learn why stability and balance are so important for the older adult population, and we will provide some exercises that can help them achieve their fitness goals.

Focusing on stability training will help you become more aware of your body's position in space, a skill known as proprioception. Reducing the likelihood of fractures and injuries caused by falls is largely dependent on this improvement. Not only does improving your balance help you prevent falls, but it also helps you improve upon the different strategies that automatically occur in situations that are "almost falls." These strategies include ankle strategy, hip strategy, and stepping strategy. Ankle strategy is the first line of defense when you lose your balance or almost fall. An example would be when you are walking uphill over a soft or compliant surface such as high grass or mud and you start to lose your balance, but the muscles around your ankles kick in and react quickly to adjust your footing and maintain your balance. Hip strategy is the next line of defense, and is a bigger movement. For example, if you are standing on a really unsteady surface and your ankle muscles kick in to stabilize you but they need more assistance, you will start to automatically hinge at the hip and move your trunk over your legs in different directions as a way to try to maintain your balance without losing your footing. If your hip strategy is unable to maintain your balance, you will automatically lose your footing and take a step, which is your "stepping strategy" kicking in to prevent you from falling. An example of this is if you're standing and someone comes and pushes you from behind. The force may cause you to lose your footing and step forward so you don't lose your balance. All of these strategies become stronger and more efficient when you consistently incorporate balance training into your fitness routine. They need to be sharpened and challenged in order to be prepared for real world scenarios.

As you improve your proprioception and sharpen your balance strategies, you start to feel more comfortable with moving freely. This facilitates increased stability and confidence in fast-paced, unsteady, and unstable environments. For example, walking uphill over grass on a busy sidewalk with a lot of cars passing by, or crossing a busy intersection with snow on the ground people walking briskly all around you. This increased freedom of mobility is imperative to allow you to feel comfortable putting your body in situations where you may have to change your walking speed often, encounter different types of terrain, walk up and down stairs or steps, or navigate large crowds of people moving in different directions. Improving your balance through working on balance and stability training has a direct correlation to your body's success in these physically challenging environments.

This boost in confidence with mobility makes people more active, which is very important for staying independent and having a good quality of life in older age. Focusing on balance and stability routines can help you live a more active, fulfilling, and safe life. As you navigate this chapter, you will learn about different balance assessments and exercises aimed at improving various components of your balance system. Access your supplemental material guide at https://bit.ly/3x3FmbJ for more information on these assessments as well as videos of the exercises.

4.2 Assessing Balance and Stability Levels

The first step to working towards improving your balance is to assess your balance and steadiness by establishing a baseline. A baseline level tells you where you stand in terms of your physical skills pertaining to balance, and shows you where you need to improve. Tests that look at your posture, standing and performing activities, gait, power, and coordination are often part of this evaluation. Once you know what you need to improve upon and identify your weaknesses, you can create goals to address them. You can also center your exercise routine around those areas.

In Chapter 2, when we discussed addressing fitness levels, we identified three balance tests which are considered evidence-based and objective outcome measures for assessing overall balance and predicting fall risk. Below we will go into more detail regarding these assessments, and then describe additional exercises and measures which may be used to effectively assess balance and stability levels. These assessments can be performed by a professional, or they can be performed on your own and used in a self-guided format to determine areas for improvement and select exercises to incorporate into your routine.

Berg Balance Scale

- Balance assessment which measures functional mobility and determines fall risk.
- Items include static and dynamic activities of varying difficulty, 14 tasks.
    - Items include sit to stand, stand to sit, static standing with eyes open and closed, transferring into/out of chair, reaching outside base of support, standing with feet together, picking up an object from the floor, weight shifting in standing, turning around, placing foot on a step stool, and standing on one leg.

BALANCE AND STABILITY EXERCISES

- Test must be performed without an assistive device; higher score is given when tasks can be performed without upper extremity support.
- Each task is scored based on performance—higher score indicates better performance.
  - Score of 45/56 or greater indicates low fall risk.

Timed Up and Go (TUG) Test

- Assesses mobility, balance, walking ability, and fall risk in older adults.
- Measures the time taken to rise from a chair, walk 3 meters, turn around, walk back, and sit down.
- May use an assistive device to perform test.
- The test is designed for someone to walk at a "quick yet safe speed" and the goal is to increase speed as balance improves.
  - Less than 13.5 seconds is considered normal and safe for a community dwelling adult.

Dynamic Gait Index (DGI)

- Assesses an individual's ability to modify balance while walking in the presence of external demands.
  - Objective is to measure walking during more challenging tasks.
- Predicts the likelihood of falling in older adults by testing 8 facets of gait.
- Items include walking on level surface, change in walking speed, walking with head turns, walking and

then suddenly stopping and turning around, stepping over obstacle while walking, stepping around obstacles, and walking up and down stairs.
- Scores are based on a 4-point scale, highest possible score is a 24—higher score indicates better performance.

These assessments can be used to guide your balance exercise program and to objectively track your progress. See below for some other simplified useful options you may use to assess your balance. Select the assessment that is most appropriate based on your current fitness level and that will highlight weak areas in order to best select exercises and create goals depending on your specific needs and lifestyle.

Single Leg Stand

- Stand on one leg while lifting the other leg slightly off the ground. Measure the duration you can maintain this position without losing your balance. This assesses static single leg balance.

Tandem Stand

- Stand with one foot in front of the other, heel to toe, in a straight line. Measure the duration you can maintain this position without losing your balance.

BALANCE AND STABILITY EXERCISES

Functional Reach Test

- Stand next to a wall and reach forward as far as possible without taking a step. Measure the distance reached. A shorter reach indicates reduced dynamic balance and stability.

Modified Clinical Test of Sensory Interaction on Balance (mCTSIB)

- Stand on a firm surface with eyes open, eyes closed, then stand on a foam or compliant surface with eyes open and eyes closed. This test evaluates how sensory input affects balance. Balance is affected by the sensation in your feet, your vision, and your vestibular system. This test helps determine which part of your balance system is weakest and needs improvement since it takes vision (eyes open/eyes closed) and sensation in your feet (firm vs compliant surface) into account.

Assessing your balance and stability is a great way to understand what areas you need to work on and select specific exercises and activities to incorporate into your fitness routine. Improving your balance and stability will allow you to feel more confident and freer in your mobility, especially in challenging and fast-paced physical situations. It is an integral part of living your best ageless fitness life.

4.3 Balance Exercises into Daily Routine

Maintaining stability and balance as you age is crucial in order to live an independent and active life. In order to sustain this independent and active life, balance exercises should be a part of your everyday regimen. These activities are very important for improving your overall physical condition, decreasing the chance of falls, and improving your coordination. It is easy and effective to incorporate these workouts into your regular routine.

Exercises for balance do not have to be difficult to include in your program. You may simply incorporate these exercises into your daily routine since they are straightforward and effective. You can practice heel-to-toe stands or standing on one foot, for example, while waiting for the coffee to brew in the kitchen or while brushing your teeth. When repeated, these minor additions to your routine can result in noticeable gains in coordination and balance. Here is how to perform the examples mentioned:

Single-Leg Stand

- Stand close to a sturdy chair or counter for support.
- Lift one leg off the ground and hold for 10-30 seconds.
- Repeat with the other leg. For a challenge, try closing your eyes.

Heel-to-Toe Walk

- Use a straight line on the floor as a guide.

- Place one foot directly in front of the other, heel touching toe.
- Walk forward a few steps, turn around, and repeat.

Integrating Exercises into Daily Activities

- While brushing your teeth, stand on one leg and switch halfway through.
- As you wait for the kettle to boil, practice standing on tiptoes to strengthen your ankles.
- Walk to/from the stove to the table performing heel-to-toe walk.

Based on the assessments performed in the previous section, you can select a few of the items that you scored lower on and were more difficult for you. Think about your daily routine, and where these items can seamlessly be performed at different, reasonable, times of the day depending on your to-do list. Then execute! Perform these activities throughout your day repeatedly. What was once a conscious thought and plan will become an automatic part of your daily routine and a habit. An advantage to incorporating these exercises into your daily routine is that you will probably discover that daily chores and tasks become easier and more pleasurable to perform. Frequent balance exercises can improve your strength and stability, which will boost your self-assurance when moving.

It is important to start with basic balance exercises and to be consistent. The best thing about these workouts is that you can incorporate them into your regular routine without needing any additional time or equipment. As you consistently perform these exercises, you will eventually reap the benefits of increased strength and stability. This improves your sense of freedom while also making daily tasks easier to handle. Thus, make the initial decision and addition to your routine, adhere to the schedule, and enjoy the improvements it makes to your day-to-day quality of life.

4.4 Stability Exercises to Improve Coordination

Coordination is crucial for maintaining good balance and for being able to react and move quickly, specifically in fast-paced environments with challenging external and environmental factors. For example, walking in the grass, snow, uphill, downhill, alongside a heavy traffic flow of people or vehicles, walking while carrying several items, having to turn in multiple directions, or having to walk around or over obstacle. These are different environmental situations we encounter in our everyday lives. The older we get, the more important it becomes to maintain and improve coordination in order to be able to safely and efficiently perform tasks and activities in different types of environments or situations.

So far, we have discussed how to assess balance, how to select specific balance exercises to address our weaknesses, and how to incorporate balance training in our everyday lives. Now we will go into more detailed and variable stability exercises that can facilitate improved overall balance and coordination. These exercises can be combined with the exercises you've selected from your balance assessments, or can be supplemental exercises to provide modifications or variability in your balance training routine.

Balloon Tap

- Stand or sit comfortably. Use a balloon and tap it gently with your hands to keep it in the air. Try to maintain a rhythmic and controlled tapping motion.

Figure-Eight Arm Swings

- Stand with feet shoulder-width apart. Extend your arms and draw a figure-eight pattern in the air with both arms simultaneously. Focus on smooth and controlled movements.

Seated Marching with Arm Crosses

- Sit in a chair with good posture. Lift one knee towards your chest while crossing the opposite arm over to touch the knee. Alternate between legs and arms in a marching motion.

Walking Patterns

- Create a walking pattern on the floor using tape or markers. Walk along the pattern, lifting knees, and turning as indicated. This helps improve coordination and spatial awareness.

Hand-Eye Coordination

- While sitting or standing, use a handheld target (i.e.: small ball or beanbag). Toss it in the air and try to catch it with your opposite hand. Increase the difficulty by varying the height and speed of the toss.

Dance or Aerobic Movements

- Participate in dance or aerobic exercises that involve coordinated movements. These classes can be taken at a studio or can be performed from the comfort of your own home through YouTube or other online video platforms.

Stability Ball Exercises

- Using a stability ball, perform various exercises that will help improve balance and coordination.
  - Seated Marching
    - Sit on the stability ball with feet flat on the floor. Lift one knee at a time towards your chest, alternating legs in a marching motion. Keep your back straight and engage your core.
  - Pelvic tilts
    - Sit on the stability ball with your feet shoulder-width apart. Slowly tilt your pelvis forward and backward, engaging your core muscles. This helps provide pelvic stability.
  - Ball squats

BALANCE AND STABILITY EXERCISES

- - Stand with the stability ball between your lower back and a wall. Lower your body into a squat position, rolling the ball down the wall. Keep your knees over your ankles and your back against the ball.
  - Standing Wall Roll
    - Stand with the ball between your back and a wall. Roll the ball up and down the wall using small movements, engaging your core. This helps improve balance and stability.

There are many different types of stability exercises, and they all focus on distinct areas of balance and coordination. The purpose of these exercises is to test and enhance your body's stability. They range from basic ones like standing on one leg to more intricate ones that incorporate several muscle groups. You will see gains in your confidence to carry out everyday tasks as well as your physical health by implementing these into your routine. As you practice these regularly, you will find that things that were once difficult become easier and safer over time. These exercises can dramatically increase your balance and coordination, lower your chance of falling, and improve your general quality of life when done with the proper form and with a customized strategy.

To get the most out of stability exercises, you must maintain a regular schedule. At least twice or three times a week, you should incorporate these workouts into your fitness routine. You can progressively push yourself by increasing the frequency and intensity of these workouts from a comfortable starting point. This method contributes significantly to boosting your general fitness and well-being in addition to improving your coordination. You will start to see changes in your movement and overall well-being as you include this program into your weekly calendar, which will help you lead a healthier, more active lifestyle.

4.5 Core Strength for Better Balance and Stability

Finding stability and balance—both necessary for leading an active and healthy lifestyle—requires having a strong core. By emphasizing core strength training, older persons can improve their quality of life in addition to their fitness. Maintaining stability is essential to preventing falls, and strengthening the core is fundamental to doing so. Beyond just bulking up your muscles, a strong core helps you maintain balance and coordination, which will make it easier and more comfortable for you to carry out daily tasks.

There are several advantages to core strength training, particularly for older adults. A strong core gives your body stability and support during all of its motions, acting as the focal point for all other body functions and movements. This stability is necessary to ensure your daily safety as well as effectiveness with performance of physical activities. You lay the groundwork for improved general health by doing workouts that strengthen your core, or the muscles surrounding your midsection, lower back, and hips. A strong core improves posture, lessens the load

BALANCE AND STABILITY EXERCISES

on your body while you move, and lowers your chance of injury, especially from balance-related problems.

Core strength essential for maintaining your balance and stability, lowering your risk of falling, and empowering you to move freely and on your own. A strong core is essential for many physical tasks, including walking, bending to tie shoes, and reaching up to high shelves. You are investing in your capacity to live an active, meaningful, and independent life far into older age when you set aside time to strengthen your core.

In Chapter 3 we discussed specific exercises that facilitate increased core strength. Here we will include additional core exercises that focus on balance and stability while strengthening the core musculature. These exercises can be performed in addition to the core exercise during strength training, or can be performed separately during your balance training exercise routine.

Marching with Torso Twist

- Stand with feet hip-width apart. Lift one knee towards your chest while simultaneously twisting your torso toward the lifted knee. Alternate legs and repeat the motion, engaging your core.

Single-Leg Balance with Arm Reach

- Stand on one leg with a slight bend in the knee. Extend one arm forward and the opposite leg backward. Hold the position for a few seconds, engaging your core for balance. Switch sides and repeat.

Plank with Leg Lift

- Start in a plank position on your hands or forearms. Lift one leg off the ground, keeping your body in a straight line. Engage your core and hold for a few seconds before switching legs. Modify by performing leg lift with one leg and maintaining stability on the opposite knee. Progress to performing in full plank position.

Seated Russian Twists

- Sit on a stability ball or chair with feet flat on the floor. Hold a ball or weight with both hands. Twist your torso to one side, then to the other, engaging your core muscles.

Standing Core Rotation

- Stand with feet hip-width apart and hold a light weight or ball with both hands. Rotate your torso to one side, then back to the center, and repeat on the other side. Keep your hips stable and engage your core throughout.

Balance Ball Roll

- Kneel on a stability ball with your hands on the floor. Slowly roll the ball forward, extending your body into a plank position. Roll the ball back towards your knees, engaging your core. Modify by keeping the range of motion smaller, to your comfort level, and progress towards full plank position as able.

Exercises such as yoga and tai chi are also excellent ways to perform balance movements and positions while engaging and strengthening the core muscles. Including these many exercise modalities in your life will improve your quality of life and help you stay active. Exercises that improve balance and strength while developing your core muscles are comprehensive and allow you to "kill two birds with one stone." Maintaining and improving balance and stability as you age requires a training regimen that heavily emphasizes core strength. This all-inclusive fitness regimen that includes a variety of workouts will keep you physically fit while also greatly improving your general health and wellness. It is an active step toward a healthier, happier, and stronger way of living.

CHAPTER 5

Low-Impact Cardio Workouts

5.1 The Benefits of Low-Impact Cardio for Older Adults

Staying active is essential to maintain health and happiness as you age. In addition to assisting with weight maintenance and lowering the risk of chronic diseases, regular exercise also has positive effects on mental health, sleep, vitality, and productivity. If you are an older adult dealing with issues like joint pain and low bone density, high-impact workouts might not be the way to go. Low-impact cardio activities are a great option and solution because they are both safe and effective.

If you suffer from arthritis or joint pain, low-impact cardio activities are ideal because they are gentle on the joints. Activities like walking, swimming, cycling, and elliptical provide a cardiovascular workout by facilitating an increase in heart rate while reducing the impact of forces through the joints.

Improved heart health is a major benefit of low-impact cardio. Aerobic exercise has several health benefits, including reducing the risk of cardiovascular disease, improving circulation, and lowering blood pressure. Raising your heart rate and breathing rate works your cardiovascular system and lungs, which improves your fitness and stamina.

Furthermore, you can alleviate joint stiffness and soreness with these mild cardiovascular workouts. These exercises can help alleviate the pain of joint caused by disorders like osteoarthritis due to the lubricating effects on the joints of repetitive motions. Being active on a regular basis increases mobility and endurance, which in turn makes carrying out everyday activities less of a chore.

Additionally, if you want to improve your stability and balance while also improving your endurance, low-impact cardiovascular exercises are a fantastic choice. Tai chi and water aerobics are great for improving balance, core strength, and coordination, while also providing aerobic benefits.

If you suffer from back pain or poor posture, try adding some low-impact cardiovascular exercise to your fitness regimen. By building stronger muscles that support the back, these exercises help to reduce strain on the spine and encourage proper spinal alignment. You can ease back pain and avoid future problems by paying close attention to your posture as you exercise. The increase in blood flow and circulation throughout your body provided by low-impact cardiovascular activity helps to loosen up the muscles, decreasing back pain and stiffness.

Finally, there are several advantages for older persons to engage in low-impact cardiovascular exercises. They are a great method to keep active and fit since they boost heart health, manage joint discomfort, improve balance and stability, and help with back pain. You may improve your health and well-being and ensure an active and satisfying life as you age by adding low-impact cardio to your training program.

5.2 Choosing Suitable Cardio Exercises

Regular cardiovascular exercise is essential for people of all ages to stay healthy. Cardio exercises have several benefits for older adults, including better heart health, increased stamina, improved mood, and overall quality of life. To maximize your workout benefits and minimize injury risk, it is essential to choose cardiovascular exercises that are suitable for your individual needs and abilities.

For older adults, low-impact workouts are ideal. You can get the cardiovascular benefits of these exercises without putting too much strain on your joints. As an example, walking is a simple kind of exercise that you can incorporate into your schedule at any time. Walking is beneficial for more than just raising your heart rate--it also aids with weight management and develops your leg muscles.

Swimming and water aerobics are great options for a low-impact cardiovascular workout that will not strain your joints. These exercises are especially helpful for people with joint discomfort or arthritis since the buoyancy of water reduces pressure and strain on the body.

An additional great low-impact cardiovascular workout is cycling, whether done outdoors or on a stationary bicycle. Riding a bike has several health benefits, including strengthening your heart and enhancing your balance, coordination, and leg strength—all of which are essential for maintaining your independence and mobility.

Exercises which provide cardiovascular benefits and are also considered functional training include yoga and tai chi. These types of exercises boost cardiovascular fitness and are great for stability, as well as improving your posture and increasing core strength. Group workouts like these are great for people of all fitness levels since they provide encouragement and camaraderie while you work out.

Pay attention to your body and ease into aerobic routines gradually. To avoid injuries, make sure your workouts always include a cool-down and warm-up. It is critical for your maximum health and well-being to choose aerobic workouts with consideration. Boost your cardiovascular health and quality of life by participating in water-based activities and low-impact workouts. Doing these cardiovascular exercises on a regular basis will put you on the road to a healthy, active lifestyle that will last a lifetime.

5.3 Cardio Workouts without Straining Joints

Living with joint pain or discomfort is a common part of aging, and it can make it hard to do standard cardio workouts. You should not let this discourage you from maintaining an active lifestyle. Many different types of low-impact cardio exercises are available in the fitness industry, which provide great options for older adults. The goal of these exercises is to keep you active and healthy without putting unnecessary strain on your joints. The design of these low-impact cardiovascular options takes into account the limitations of conventional cardio equipment while still providing the health advantages of cardiovascular exercise, such as increased heart rate, enhanced endurance, and general well-being, without the risk of injury to the joints.

The beauty of these low-impact exercises is that they provide new opportunities to be physically active and keep your heart rate up without putting unnecessary stress on your joints. When it comes to age-related problems like arthritis or common wear and tear on the joints, low-impact cardio activities are a great method to maintain mobility without risking injury. As you face the inevitable changes that come with becoming older, they make sure that you may keep your health and fitness as top priorities.

Below we outline specific exercises which should be performed as low-impact options to preserve joint integrity.

Swimming

- Offers a full-body workout.

LOW-IMPACT CARDIO WORKOUTS

- Water buoyancy supports body weight, reducing joint impact.
- Options include swimming laps, water aerobics, or water walking/jogging.

Cycling

- Can be done on a stationary bike or traditional bicycle.
- Provides excellent cardiovascular exercise with minimal joint stress.
- Resistance levels can be adjusted to suit your fitness level.

Elliptical

- Gentle on the joints while offering increases in circulation and heart rate.

Rowing Machine

- A low-impact option that also provides strength training benefits.

Stationary Marching

- Can be performed sitting or standing.
- Offers core strengthening and balance benefits while also increasing heart rate.
- Can be adjusted and modified based on fitness levels by increasing or decreasing speed and duration.

Tai Chi and Yoga

- Low-impact, provides combination multi-directional and multi-joint movements.
- Provides balance, flexibility, and core strength benefits.
- Combines gentle movements and deep breathing.

Dancing

- Enjoyable and can provide mental health and mood enhancing benefits.
- Can perform in group setting.
- Full-body and low-impact cardio benefits, as well as coordination benefits.

Step Aerobics with Low Step Height

- Engages cardiovascular system, strengthens leg muscles, and improves balance.

It is essential to pay attention to your body's signals when starting an exercise program, particularly as you get older. Take it easy at first and pay close attention to your body for signs of pain. It is critical to include a cool-down period following your workout and a warm-up period before you begin. Following these guidelines can greatly reduce the likelihood of injury and ensure that your training routine remains both effective and pleasant.

These low-impact workouts are great because they address your body's specific demands while still giving you the cardiovascular advantages your body needs. You may be proactive about your health and maintaining your vitality by regularly engaging in these low-impact activities.

Maintaining a healthy lifestyle in older age requires regular activity, especially joint-friendly forms of exercise like low-impact cardio. In addition to assisting with physical fitness, it promotes general wellness.

5.4 Modifying Intensity and Duration of Cardio Workouts

Cardiovascular exercise is key in maintaining a healthy heart, managing weight, and boosting overall endurance. As an older adult, it's critical to tailor the intensity and duration of your cardio workouts for optimal safety and effectiveness.

Here's how you can adapt your cardio routines to align with your needs and capabilities, whether you're a seasoned exercise enthusiast or just starting out on your fitness journey.

Focus on Low-Impact Exercises

- Choose activities like walking, swimming, cycling, and water aerobics.
- These exercises are gentle on the joints yet provide excellent cardiovascular benefits.

Incorporate Diverse Fitness Elements

- Add strength training, balance and stability exercises, functional training, and posture improvement into your routine.
- These elements enhance overall fitness and promote joint health and fall prevention.

Managing Joint Pain Through Exercise

- Engage in activities that strengthen muscles around your joints, reducing discomfort.
- Implement proper techniques to alleviate joint pain and enhance your quality of life.

Adjust Intensity and Duration

- Find the right balance that challenges you without overexertion.
- Determine and monitor your target heart rate zone for appropriate exercise intensity.
- Gradually increase and vary the duration of workouts to continuously challenge your body safely.

Specifically, when it comes to intensity, follow these guidelines to appropriately customize your cardiovascular training program :

Moderate Intensity

- Aim for a moderate intensity, where you can still carry on a conversation but feel slightly breathless.

- Use the "talk test": if you can talk comfortably during the exercise, it's likely at a moderate intensity.

Perceived Exertion

- Use the Rate of Perceived Exertion (RPE) scale from 1 to 10. Aim for an RPE of around 5 or 6, where 1 is very light activity, and 10 is maximal effort.

Heart Rate

- Aim for around 50-70% of your maximum heart rate. The formula for calculating your maximum heart rate is 220 minus your age.

For modifying duration and adjusting your cardiovascular workouts to your specific needs and capabilities, follow these guidelines:

Start Slow

- Begin with shorter bouts of duration and gradually increase over time. You can perform several short bouts in one session if that is a more comfortable way to start. For example, perform 3 bouts of 5 minutes of elliptical training with 2-3 minutes of rest in between each bout.
- Start with about 10-15 minutes of cumulative cardio per session and progress to 30 minutes per session.

Frequency

- Aim for at least 150 minutes of moderate intensity aerobic activity per week. This can be spread throughout the week, with the goal being about 30 minutes on most days.

Incremental Increases

- Once comfortable with a certain duration, gradually increase the time spent on cardio exercises in small increments, such as 2-5 minutes per bout or session.

Consistency

- Consistency is key. Regular, shorter workouts are more beneficial than sporadic, longer sessions.

In order to maximize the benefits of cardiovascular exercise without risking injuries or overstressing your body it is crucial to know how to adjust the intensity and duration of your exercises. You can tailor your exercise routine to your specific demands and abilities by varying the intensity and duration of your workouts. These modifications can be changed as you progress through your ageless fitness journey or as your health circumstances change. With this approach, you can prioritize your wellness by keeping your heart healthy, controlling your weight successfully, and increasing your stamina.

You can improve your health by pushing yourself to your limits, but you can also learn to listen to your body and adjust your aerobic routine accordingly. The key is to achieve a balance between feeling overly fatigued or causing an injury, and the exercise feeling too easy. With this comprehensive method, you may enjoy the many benefits of cardiovascular exercise while also meeting your body where it is in every moment. The goal is to lead an active and fruitful life and feel confident in knowing that your exercise regimen is beneficial, but also safe and appropriate for your specific needs.

5.5 Creating a Varied and Enjoyable Cardio Routine

As you get older, cardiovascular activity is an important part of maintaining health and fitness. Regular cardio activities are important for keeping your heart healthy, building stamina, and feeling more energized in general. However, it can be hard for many older people to find fitness activities that they enjoy and that do not cause discomfort or pain. The goal is to create a varied and fun cardio routine that works for you and fits seamlessly into your weekly routine.

First, it is important to choose workouts that align with your fitness level, especially if you have any health problems or joint pain. Walking, swimming, cycling, or water aerobics are all examples of low-impact activities that can be started, modified, and progressed at any fitness level. These exercises are good for your joints and still give your heart and lungs a good workout.

Try doing different things every day of the week to keep your mode of cardio training interesting and new. For example, you could plan to go for a fast walk in the park one day, swim the next, and go on a scenic bike ride with friends on the weekend. This variety not only keeps things exciting, but it also encourages working out a lot of different muscle groups, which makes exercise more beneficial.

Taking a group fitness class for older people can make your routine more social and fun. In these classes, you might do aerobic dance, tai chi, or movements in a chair. Not only do they help your heart health, but they also give you a chance to meet new people and provide entertainment with a group.

Another important aspect to creating a variable and enjoyable cardiovascular training routine is to set goals that are attainable. Begin your workout journey with shorter workouts and work your way up to longer ones. Aim for at least 150 minutes of moderate aerobic exercise per week, or 75 minutes if you prefer more intense activities and can handle them safely. Be consistent with your routine. Feeling like you set a goal and achieve it each week creates a positive effect that leads to increased motivation and overall compliance. This creates a habit and a lifestyle change.

Designing a fun and varied exercise routine is important for keeping your heart healthy and staying fit as you get older. You can formulate your own cardio routine that keeps you busy, motivated, and healthy as you get older by choosing low-impact exercises, changing up your routine, joining group classes, setting goals that you can reach, and paying attention to your body and its evolving needs.

CHAPTER 6

Joint Pain Management Through Exercise

6.1 Common Joint Pain Issues in Older Adults

Joint pain is a frequent problem that many people have as they become older. It can have a substantial influence on your quality of life as well as your capacity to continue being active and independent. In this chapter, we will discuss typical joint pain concerns that older persons experience and lead you toward effectively managing these problems through the inclusion of exercise and lifestyle adaptations.

Arthritis is the most common cause of joint discomfort in people who are older. As the protective cartilage that cushions your joints wears away over time, osteoarthritis, the most common kind, develops. This condition causes pain, stiffness, and a reduction in movement. Rheumatoid arthritis is another type of arthritis that is rather common and is characterized by inflammation and pain in the joints. Gout is another form of arthritis that is characterized by the buildup of uric acid crystals in the joints, leading to sudden and severe pain, swelling, and redness, often affecting the big toe.

Tendonitis is another common cause of joint pain. It is defined by inflammation or irritation of a tendon, the thick cord that attaches muscles to bones. It commonly occurs in the shoulders, elbows, knees, and heels, causing pain and tenderness. It can occur as a result of overuse of muscles and tendons, from repetitive motions, incorrect form or posture during mobility or exercise, and increase strain put on the tendon during exercise. Strength training with correct form is imperative in order to assist in the prevention of tendonitis.

Degenerative disc disease is frequently seen in adults as we age. It primarily affects the spine, and can lead to pain in the facet joints of the spine, causing discomfort and reduced mobility. Maintaining proper spinal alignment and posture is a very important part of slowing down and preventing degenerative disc disease. Spinal stenosis is defined as the narrowing of spaces within the spine, which can put pressure on the nerves. This can lead to pain, weakness, and/or numbness in the arms or legs. Consistent work on posture and mobility helps maintain proper spinal alignment and prevent stenosis.

Another common issue that affects older adults and can cause joint issues and pain is osteoporosis. Osteoporosis is a condition characterized by weakened bones, making them more susceptible to fractures. Fractures can cause joint pain and affect mobility, and should be prevented by all means possible.

Carpal tunnel syndrome results from compression of the median nerve as it passes through the carpal tunnel in the wrist. It is caused by repetitive, overuse wrist motion over time, such as typing. It causes pain, numbness, and tingling in the wrist and hand. Keeping the wrist in a neutral position (a wrist splint/brace may help), an ergonomic work station, and addressing any symptoms of pain right away as they appear are crucial for preventing carpal tunnel syndrome from developing into a debilitating issue.

Bursitis is another condition that can cause joint pain and discomfort, as well as swelling. It is the inflammation of the fluid-filled sacs (bursae) that cushion and reduce friction between bones, tendons, and muscles. It is imperative to create and maintain strength, stability, and range of motion around the joint to reduce the chances of increased stress and inflammation in these areas.

Meniscus tears are common due to wear and tear or injury. The meniscus is a cartilage in the knee that protects the joint. A tear in this cartilage can cause pain, swelling, and difficulty moving the knee. Strengthening the leg muscles around the knee and working on a balance program to ensure multi-directional movements are performed safely is a vital component to maintaining the integrity of the meniscus and preventing injury which can lead to pain and decreased mobility.

Knowledge about these common issues causing joint pain in older adults is essential in order to understand what course to take to prevent these issues and to remain proactive about early treatment of any symptoms that may arise. The good news is that living an ageless fitness lifestyle consisting of exercise, diet, and proper recovery is the best medicine which will help combat these issues as we age and become more susceptible to them.

6.2 The Role of Exercise in Managing Joint Pain

Exercise can play a significant part in controlling and even lowering the discomfort that is associated with joint pain, which becomes increasingly more prevalent with age. There are several ways in which physical activity assists in alleviating joint discomfort, increasing fitness, and boosting quality of life.

Physical activity can provide tremendous relief to anyone living with joint discomfort and pain. Unless you are dealing with a specific condition where exercise is contraindicated or you have specific exercise restrictions that have been provided from a medical professional, exercising at a comfortable level will typically benefit you and provide relief. When you engage in regular physical exercise, the muscles that surround your joints become stronger, which provides more support and stability. Your joints will experience less tension as a result of this, which will result in less discomfort and improved mobility.

Strength training can be very beneficial for those suffering from joint pain. Strength training techniques that involve resistance, such as lifting weights or utilizing resistance bands, are beneficial for developing muscle strength and improving joint stability. You will experience less discomfort as a result of this, and it will also enhance your overall physical function and lower the likelihood that you may fall, leading to further joint pain or problems.

An additional essential component of joint pain management is the use of exercises that focus on balance and stability. Performing these exercises can help you improve your coordination and proprioception, both of which are essential for avoiding falls and improving your stability. One can considerably improve their balance and lessen the likelihood of sustaining joint injuries by engaging in activities such as standing on one leg or using a balance board.

When it comes to managing joint discomfort, low-impact aerobics routines are essential. Walking, swimming, and cycling are examples of activities that are beneficial to your cardiovascular system without putting an excessive amount of stress on your joints. These exercises contribute to an improvement in circulation, a reduction in inflammation, and an overall improvement in joint health.

Functional training is necessary for elderly people who are experiencing joint pain. Squats and lunges are two examples of exercises that replicate daily activities. These exercises improve strength and mobility, which in turn makes it easier to perform daily duties, reducing joint discomfort and strain.

The adjustment of posture and the performance of exercises to alleviate back pain are also vital. Having poor posture can make joint pain even more severe and cause additional suffering due to muscle asymmetries and malalignment. One way to alleviate back discomfort and improve posture, which in turn reduces stress on the joints, is to concentrate on exercises that strengthen the core and improve spinal alignment.

Physical activity is an essential component in the management of joint pain in older persons. You can find significant relief from joint discomfort by engaging in activities such as strengthening exercises, exercises that enhance balance, low-impact aerobics, functional training, and correcting your posture. When it comes to the management of joint pain and overall well-being, it is never too late to begin exercising and gain the myriad of benefits that physical activity provides.

6.3 Incorporating Joint-Friendly Exercises into Fitness Routine

Focusing on joint health and maintaining overall fitness becomes increasingly critical as you advance in age. Engaging in regular exercise tailored to your needs can significantly enhance various aspects of your health, including strength, flexibility, balance, and stability. The key lies in choosing the right kind of exercises that are gentle on your joints while effectively contributing to your long-term health and well-being.

When you exercise with a focus on joint health, you're not just working out--you're investing in your future ability to stay active and independent. The goal is to find those exercises that fortify your body without causing unnecessary strain or risk to your joints. This intentional selection of exercises ensures that each workout contributes positively to your overall fitness, helping to build a body that's strong, flexible, and balanced. By incorporating joint-friendly routines into your exercise regimen, you are taking a proactive step towards maintaining a high quality of life and overall well-being.

This strategy of incorporating joint-friendly exercises into your routine safely allows you to enhance your strength, ensuring you have the muscle power to perform daily tasks effortlessly. It also increases flexibility, allowing your body to move freely and comfortably. It improves your balance, reducing the risk of falls and injuries, and it boosts your overall stability, giving you the confidence to navigate your day with ease. All of these benefits come together to ensure that as you age, your fitness routine continues to support a vibrant, active, ageless fitness lifestyle.

Based on the different types of exercises recommended to include in your ageless fitness routine, here is how you can seamlessly incorporate joint-friendly choices into each mode/category of your fitness routine:

Strength Training

- Use lighter weights or resistance bands for resistance exercises.
- Perform bodyweight exercises such as squats, lunges, wall push-ups, tricep dips at the edge of a chair, etc.
- Perform seated strengthening such as marches or leg lifts in a stable chair.

- If at a gym or exercise facility, use selectorized resistance training machines that have handles, seats, and back support in order to isolate the muscle being trained and ensure proper form and support of your body while performing the movements.
- These options build muscle mass, crucial for supporting your joints, without putting excessive strain on them.

Balance and Stability Exercises

- Always perform balance and stability exercises near a stable surface to hold onto with your arms for safety, such as a chair or counter.
- Gradually progress from firm to more compliant surfaces to avoid overly stressing or twisting the ankle and knee joints while working on balance training and balance recovery exercises.
- Perform all exercises with arm support for a few repetitions first, then gradually take away upper extremity support.
- Gradually include some of the easier to moderate balance exercises into your daily routine to facilitate as much repetition as possible, therefore decreasing the fall/injury risk as your body and balance system adjust.
- Incorporate yoga poses, such as the tree pose, or tai chi movements, to enhance your stability while also working on flexibility, which decreases strain on the joints.

Low-Impact Cardio Workouts

- Opt for activities like walking, swimming, cycling, or using an elliptical machine.
- Start with low to moderate intensity, based on your fitness level, and gradually increase.
- Take group aerobic classes which are tailored to senior/older adults—they will focus on keeping all of the movements safe and joint-friendly.
- Water aerobics is an excellent option to provide resistance without impact.
- Perform your cardio in intervals and take appropriate breaks and perform stretching in between—listen to your body.
- Avoid high-impact movements such as jumping or running.
- These workouts are easy on the joints while still providing cardiovascular benefits.

Flexibility

- Engage in exercises that enhance joint mobility and flexibility, like gentle stretching, yoga, and tai chi.
- Be consistent and target all major muscle groups with flexibility training.
- Use a heating pad to increase circulation if you are stretching at home and your muscles are not warmed up.
- Most people wake up feeling stiff, which worsens as you age. Incorporate light, full-body stretches in your morning routine prior to starting your activities for

the day to facilitate joint movement and flexibility and prevent injury.
- These activities can alleviate stiffness and pain, helping you maintain an active lifestyle.

Functional Training

- Focus on exercises that simulate everyday movements, such as squats, lunges, overhead press, lateral raises, sitting up from lying on your back, sit to stands, etc.
- Target all major muscle groups and focus on compound movements which use multiple muscle groups for one movement. This helps distribute the force used by each muscle group, decreasing the demand on one specific joint.
- Perform movements through their full range of motion. This preserves overall range, so that if one day you perform an activity/movement that you don't perform often, your joints are prepared to move through a full range and it is not a foreign range of motion for them.
- This training improves your strength and mobility for daily tasks, keeping you physically prepared for life's demands as you age.

Posture Improvement and Back Pain Relief

- Postural awareness is important. Daily postural checks and incorporating simple, quick, postural exercises into your everyday routine will prevent excess strain on the joints through repetitive, misaligned, prolonged

positioning from bad posture. For example, shoulder rolls, shoulder blade squeezes, chin tucks, and abdominal tucks/pelvic tilts.
- Sleeping position is crucial to prevent excess strain on joints for a prolonged period of time throughout the night. Some tips that can promote better posture during sleep are: sleeping with a pillow in between your legs if on your side or under your knees if on your back, adjusting pillow height under your head depending on your position, sleeping on a firmer mattress, and frequent changing or flipping of your mattress.
- Strengthen your core and back muscles with exercises like planks, bridges, and bird-dog.
- Adjust work or computer station to ensure that it is ergonomically friendly. This includes height and distance of screen, chair adjustments, keyboard and arm positioning while typing, and frequent standing rest breaks.
- These exercises improve posture and help alleviate back pain, contributing to better joint health.

Implementing these considerations in your fitness routine will help your joints stay healthy over time, make you more stable, as well as help to alleviate and manage existing joint pain.

6.4 Stretching and Flexibility Exercises for Joint Pain Relief

Joint pain is a common issue as you get older, often due to arthritis, past injuries, or the natural aging process. This pain can significantly affect your daily life and mobility. But there's a silver lining: adding stretching and flexibility exercises to your fitness routine can offer substantial joint pain relief and improve joint function over time.

Stretching exercises are vital, especially for older adults. They enhance flexibility, improve your range of motion, and ease muscle tension, which in turn helps alleviate joint pain. Regularly including stretching in your routine boosts your physical performance and supports an active lifestyle.

Stretching should occur daily, if possible. It is safe to stretch at any time, but may be beneficial to stretch in the morning when your body typically feels stiffer and tighter. When stretching surrounding a workout, it is best to perform prolonged stretches after the workout. You should stretch all major muscle groups, but make sure to focus on stretches that target areas affected by joint pain and the specific muscle groups exercised during that workout session. Each stretch should be held for one full minute at end-range. It may feel slightly uncomfortable if your muscles are tight, but should not feel extremely uncomfortable or painful.

Some effective stretching exercises for joint pain relief to include in your ageless fitness regimen are outlined below. Access your supplemental material resource at https://bit.ly/3x3FmbJ for video demonstrations of the stretches discussed in this section.

Neck Stretch

- Gently tilt your head to one side, bringing your ear toward your shoulder.
- Apply overpressure at the top of your head with the hand on the same side that your head is leaning toward, bringing your head down a little more toward your shoulder.
- Bring your opposite shoulder down, away from your ear at the same time to ensure better results and muscle lengthening.

Shoulder and Upper Back Stretch

- Stand tall, extend one arm across your chest.
- Use your other hand to gently pull it closer.

Chest Opener Stretch

- Clasp your hands behind your back and straighten your arms.
- Lift your arms slightly, while squeezing your shoulder blades together.

Wrist and Forearm Stretch

- Extend your arm with your palm facing down. Use your opposite hand to gently press down on your fingers.
- Alternate direction and use your opposite hand to gently pull your fingers back toward your body.

Hip Flexor Stretch

- Step forward into a lunge position, keeping your back leg straight. Sink into the stretch, feeling in the hip flexor (in the hip bend/crease between your upper thigh and your abdomen) of the back leg.

Quadriceps Stretch

- Stand by a wall or chair for balance.
- Bend one knee, grasp your ankle, and gently pull your heel towards your buttock.

Hamstring Stretch

- Sit on the edge of a chair with one leg extended.
- Keep your back straight, lean forward from your hips until you feel a stretch in the back of your thigh.

Inner Thigh Stretch

- Sit in a butterfly position with your knees bent and feet together OR with your legs extended to the sides and your knees straight (whichever is more comfortable).

- Lean forward, reaching away from your body as far as you feel comfortable. You should feel a stretch on the inside of your thighs.

Outer Thigh and Glute Stretch

- Sit with one leg extended and one knee bent and crossed over the extended leg.
- Hug the bent knee with the arm on the same side, bringing it up toward your chest.
- Gently twist your torso toward that knee.

Calf Stretch

- Face a wall, hands at shoulder height on the wall.
- Step one foot back, keep it straight with the heel down.
- Lean forward slightly for a calf stretch.

Spinal Twist Stretch

- Lie on your back with both knees bent and feet flat on the floor.
- Extend your arms to the side, in a T-shape with palms facing down.
- Bring one knee toward your chest and cross it over the opposite leg, while trying to keep both shoulders on the ground.
- Gently twist your lower body to bring the crossed knee toward the floor on the opposite side.

- Turn your head in the opposite direction of the knee to look over your shoulder in order to deepen the stretch.

Remember to perform all stretches on both sides of the body. Breathe deeply and relax into each stretch. Avoid any movements that cause pain and gradually build up the range of motion and duration of your stretches as your flexibility improves.

6.5 Using Proper Form and Technique to Prevent Joint Strain

Being fit and healthy as you get older means protecting your joints also becomes more important. You may greatly lessen the likelihood of straining or injuring your joints by learning and using the correct form and technique when exercising. Let us explore many approaches to guarantee maximal benefits during your exercise regimen while emphasizing the maintenance of healthy joints.

Strength Training

Correct form is key in strength training. Maintaining proper body alignment includes having a neutral spine, shoulders back and down, and a stable core. Perform exercises with controlled and deliberate movements, avoiding momentum. Breathe consistently and avoid holding your breath. Inhale during the easier phase of the exercise, and exhale during the more challenging phase (exertion). Use a full range of motion for each exercise, moving the joints through their complete range.

Avoid overarching or rounding the back during exercises. Wear supportive footwear to provide stability and reduce the risk of injury. Use mirrors as visual cues for feedback to ensure proper form.

Balance and Stability

These exercises are crucial for improving coordination, reducing fall risks, and strengthening muscles around your joints. To prevent joint strain and ensure safety, perform balance exercises in a safe environment, free of obstacles. Use a sturdy chair or a countertop for support if needed. When practicing balance exercises, focus on keeping your alignment correct and your weight distribution even. Keep your knees slightly bent, maintaining a "soft" rather than locked position. This helps absorb shock and provides better stability. Choose a fixed point in front of you to focus on during exercises. This helps improve concentration and balance. Perform movements in a controlled manner. Avoid rapid or jerky motions, as these can compromise stability. Consider practicing some balance exercises barefoot to engage the muscles in your feet and enhance proprioception.

Low-Impact Cardio

Engaging in low-impact cardio is ideal for minimizing joint stress. It is imperative to wear proper footwear, consisting of closed, supportive, and comfortable athletic shoes that provide cushioning and stability. Choose exercise that allow for gentle, low-impact movements. Use machines that provide support such as handles and stable footplates. Maintain a neutral spine and upright posture—stand or walk tall, with your shoulders back and down, engaging your core muscles. Incorporate gentle arm movements to support good posture and balance, as well as to enhance cardiovascular benefits. Focus on controlled and rhythmic breathing. Inhale through your nose and exhale through your mouth. Be mindful of your body's signals and steer clear of activities that aggravate joint pain or are high-impact.

Functional Training

Exercises that mimic everyday activities enhance your ability to perform daily tasks efficiently and safely. Using proper form and technique is especially important during functional training exercises because these are the movements that you are more than likely to reproduce throughout the day, outside of your workout routine. Therefore, avoiding bad body mechanics and posture during these exercises is crucial for maintaining joint integrity. It is imperative to maintain a neutral spine and good posture while performing these movements, especially because a lot of these movements are considered compound movements, meaning they involve multiple joints and multiple directions. If not performed properly, these movements may pose a higher risk of injury due to the involvement of multiple joints and multiple directions at one time. It is important to keep your head up, chin tucked, shoulders back and down, and engage your core muscles. Use controlled movements, maintain stable foot placement, and breathe consistently. Go through the full range of motion, without discomfort, and gradually increase range of motion as flexibility improves. Start by performing part of the motion, then add on parts of the motion after a few repetitions, if performing a complex movement—i.e.: a squat to overhead press. If adding weight or any type of resistance, keep the weight close to your body, and use your legs to lead any heavy lifting—hinge at the hip and bend your knees. Avoid a C-shaped or curved back at all times.

Posture Matters

Poor posture can strain your joints and lead to back pain. Include exercises in your routine that strengthen your core and enhance upright postural alignment. This not only improves your posture, but also alleviates back pain.

As you get older, it becomes increasingly important to use the right form and technique when you work out. Maintaining your fitness and keeping your joints healthy are both benefits to prioritizing proper form and technique during exercise. Remember to always pay attention to your body and make changes as required. For example, modifying or adjusting weight, range of motion, or repetitions of exercises. Maintaining proper form and technique is a priority for long-term joint preservation and safety. Creating the habit of practicing proper form, technique, and postural alignment during exercise and in your daily routine is the key to enjoying the long-lasting benefits of pain-free, healthy joints in older adulthood.

CHAPTER 7

Functional Training for Daily Activities

7.1 The Importance of Functional Training in Older Adults

Sustaining an active and self-sufficient lifestyle requires maintaining strength, balance, and overall fitness. Exercises that replicate common daily actions like bending, lifting, reaching, and walking are the main focus of functional training. Enhancing your quality of life by increasing your capacity to carry out these tasks with ease and efficiency is the aim.

Exercises that target numerous muscular groups simultaneously, called compound movements, help you increase strength and range of motion. Examples of these exercises are: squats, lunges, push-ups, deadlifts, bicep curls to overhead press, etc. These exercises simulate movements that are performed in everyday tasks such as sitting, standing, reaching, getting out of bed, cleaning, etc. When you incorporate these functional training movements into your fitness routine, you perform several repetitions and add resistance, hence making the exercise a more advanced and difficult version of the task you are simulating. This, in turn, allows the functional task to feel "easier" and be performed more automatically and seamlessly relative to the training task. Functional strength training is a very task-specific way of improving your everyday quality of life and sustaining the ability to perform high-level, active tasks as you get older.

Functional training exercises are excellent for enhancing stability and balance. Since a lot of functional movements involve moving in different directions, different speeds, and with varying degrees of leg support, they naturally involve challenging your balance. For example, walking up and down stairs, stepping up onto a curb, walking up a hill, walking over snow or unlevel dirt, crossing a busy street, etc. When you work on balance exercises selected from certain outcome measures, such as the Dynamic Gait Index, for example, it challenges you to perform these functional movements in a safe, controlled, and repetitive fashion. This allows you to work on improving your balance, targeting your weaknesses. The goal is to be able to then carry over that balance training of functional movements into the real world, feeling safer and more confident as you navigate challenging, fast-paced environments.

Another important benefit of functional training is its low-impact nature. The goal of functional training is to directly improve your ability to carry out daily tasks. Therefore, for older adults, this should involve low-impact activities and exercises simulating everyday tasks. When performed repetitively, these exercises can provide a cardiovascular training effect, and as a result, improve one's endurance in the real world. For example, if you train with an aerobic step, performing step ups continually for 5 minutes, you will feel a cardiovascular training effect, and will most likely feel less winded or fatigued when walking up a flight of stairs at home or in the community. This depicts an improvement in endurance and is directly correlated to performing functional tasks repetitively. Tests such as the "Six-Minute Walk Test", which we discussed previously in Chapter 2, can be utilized as a method for functional training in your exercise routine. If you perform the test as an exercise and monitor improvement over time, you will notice that the practice and repetition will afford an increase in walking speed and endurance. This cardiovascular training effect will carry over into everyday tasks, allowing you to feel like you can walk further and faster with less fatigue when walking in the community.

Functional training can help relieve back discomfort and enhance posture if performed consistently and correctly. By incorporating repetitive functional movements during an exercise routine, you are establishing movement patterns within your brain and spine circuitry which, when done with correct form and technique, facilitate repetitive core and postural muscle activation. Over time, you are creating a training effect which promotes use of the core and postural muscles. This training will carry over into performing daily tasks with the core engaged and postural muscles activated, which leads to relief of back pain and improvement with overall posture. An example to depict this concept is sweeping. If someone who does not work out or incorporate functional training exercises into their routine sweeps, they are likely going to have a C-shaped, rounded back, their core muscles will be disengaged, and therefore they will have excess strain on their low back muscles, leading to back pain and their body being used to poor posture. However, if someone who consistently works out and performs functional training exercises in their routine is sweeping, their body is conditioned and prepared to use the correct movement patterns and muscles to perform this task. This person will have their core muscles engaged, shoulders back, spine in a neutral and upright position, and therefore much less strain forces on their low back muscles. This person's body is much more equipped for living out an active, pain-free lifestyle, and sustaining this lifestyle into older adulthood.

Functional training is an integral part of fitness, especially in older adulthood. Establishing positive movement patterns through repetition of these exercises creates a snowball effect of useful habits which facilitate living a pain-free ageless fitness lifestyle.

7.2 Identifying Functional Fitness Goals for Daily Activities

Maintaining mobility and ability in daily life requires concentrating on functional fitness objectives designed specifically for older individuals. These objectives should be age appropriate, and also be tailored to your specific daily routine, lifestyle, environment, abilities, and goals.

FUNCTIONAL TRAINING FOR DAILY ACTIVITIES

The core of functional fitness is training that mimics everyday activities. By focusing on the muscles and motions required for daily activities, you will increase your strength, stability, balance, and endurance. This method reduces the danger of falls and injuries while also making tasks like carrying groceries, getting out bed, or getting up from a low chair easier to accomplish.

The assessments outlined in Chapter 2 can help guide the selection of exercises to incorporate into your functional training routine. As you score the assessments and identify challenging or weak areas, select those items and perform them as exercises. This safe repetition of difficult tasks will translate into improved performance of daily activities and overall fitness levels. As you reassess your fitness levels using these assessments, continue to change your functional training routine, sticking to the exercises that are more challenging. For example, if you scored low on the Timed Up and Go test (TUG), pick apart the tasks in the test, and perform them individually in your exercise routine. This could mean walking a short distance and quickly turning around to walk back, and turning that into an exercise of 10 repetitions as quickly and safely as possible. Following that, you could perform sit to stands for 30 seconds, as many repetitions as possible, and repeat that 3 times. This is an example of incorporating different components of an assessment into your functional training routine, with the goal being to score higher on the assessment the next time you test, as well as improving upon tasks you perform daily such as sitting, standing, walking, and turning.

You could work on balancing on an inclined wedge and perform different exercises on it for dynamic stability, and also find a less steep incline in your community to walk up and down for a certain number of repetitions. You could then work on step ups without using your arms for a certain amount of time or repetitions. Practicing these tasks will undoubtedly improve your ability to perform your desired goal with greater ease and confidence. An example of an activity you may want to do but feel like you can't is getting onto the floor to play with your grandchild. You may start with using a surface for upper extremity support and working on a lunge transition down to your knees, and then onto the floor, and practice each of those steps several times. You can then practice transitioning back to both knees, then a lunge, and use your arms to get back up to a standing or sitting position. You can also work on performing the task without arm support as you feel more confident with your flexibility, strength, and balance. Breaking this one task into several small parts and practicing them over time will result in you eventually being able to perform the desired end-goal. The key is to identify your functional goals based on your daily routine and safely perform the parts or entire task until you achieve your goal.

Some functional training goals for older adults that target common daily activities are:

- Walking and mobility
- Stair climbing
- Rising from a chair
- Lifting and carrying groceries
- Reaching and stretching
- Bending and stooping

- Getting in and out of bed
- Cooking and meal preparation
- Personal care activities
- Opening heavy doors and handling small objects (i.e.: opening jars, etc.)
- Balancing while dressing
- Getting in and out of a car
- Getting in and out of a bath tub
- Using public transportation
- Gardening or doing yard work
- Participating in social activities
- Playing with grandchildren
- Household chores

This list is meant to help spark ideas for functional training goals that pertain to your specific lifestyle. Preserving your independence and general well-being as an older adult requires that you develop functional fitness goals that are unique to your needs. You can improve your daily life and ensure a more active and meaningful day to day experience as you age by incorporating functional training exercises into your routine.

7.3 Functional Exercises into Fitness Program

For older adults, these functional workouts are crucial. They offer an effective and practical method of conditioning your body for the tasks you encounter on a daily basis by intentionally imitating the motions and demands of such activities. With regular practice, this type of exercise will make even the most mundane tasks, like carrying groceries or navigating your home, much less of a chore. This targeted workout program is great for your physical health, but it is also important for keeping your independence and enjoying life more abundantly.

Here's how we recommend you incorporate these exercises into your fitness program:

Assessment and Selection

- Based on the assessments discussed in Chapter 2 and in section 7.2 of this chapter, select purposeful exercises which you can safely perform, but seem challenging.
- Select an appropriate number of exercises based on how many days per week and how much time each day you intend to incorporate these exercises.
- As a starting point, we recommend you select 5-10 exercises, and spend either 30 min 1-2 days/week or 10-15 min 3-4 days/week working on these in conjunction with your other exercises in your routine.
- As long as you're warmed up, it is safe to perform these exercises either before or after your strength training, balance, cardio, or postural exercises. It may provide benefits to your body to vary when you perform these exercises in your routine. Some days perform them before you're fatigued from other exercises, and some days perform them after. This mimics a more realistic simulation of when you would perform these tasks in your real-world routine.

Set Clear Goals

- As mentioned in section 7.2, it is important to tailor your functional routine to your specific needs and abilities. Setting clear and specific goals is also important.
- Identify exact activities you want to improve or be able to perform.
- Define a current measurable level of difficulty. For example, use a scale of 0-5, 0 being you cannot currently perform the task, and 5 being it is easy to perform.
- Break up the task, if necessary, into part-task components. Perform for a certain number of sets and repetitions, or for a certain amount of time. This rep scheme can be similar to how you prescribe your other modes of exercise, such as 3 sets x 10-15 reps or bouts of 3-5 minutes with short breaks in between.
- Identify a realistic timeframe in which you want to perform the task at a certain difficulty level (0-5). Perform the task in your fitness routine for a set amount of time (about 2-3 months, depending on the frequency), and then re-assess the task and difficulty level.
- Remove and add different tasks as appropriate after re-assessment. Once you feel like you no longer need to work on the task as an exercise and can safely perform it to your set goal/standard, you can replace that task with another one.

Warm-Up

- Ensure you are warmed up prior to performing your functional training exercises. These exercises can be performed in any order in your fitness routine, but should always be performed after the warm-up.

Use Bodyweight and Functional Tools

- Start with bodyweight exercises and gradually incorporate functional tools such as resistance bands, stability balls, and light weights to add resistance and variety.

Progress Gradually

- Progress the intensity and complexity of exercises gradually. Begin with foundational movements and increase difficulty as you become more comfortable and gain strength, balance, coordination, and flexibility.

Adapt to Individual Needs and Fitness Program

- Include functional training strategically into your current fitness routine. These exercises should supplement your existing program, and should be scheduled in an intentional fashion.
- Considerations include: duration of workout, type of other exercises performing that day, daily routine and physical demands of other activities outside of workout that day, difficulty level of functional training exercise, compatibility of functional training exercises with other types of exercises, your body's current state that day or week.

- For example: if you have plans to visit your daughter who lives up a steep hill with 4 steps to enter her home in the afternoon, and are going to work out that morning, it may be a good idea to practice the balance exercises on the wedge for stability, and then perform a light set of sit to stands without weights. This will train the movements you are going to use to get to your daughter's house, while preventing fatigue and muscle soreness. In this example, fatigue and muscle soreness may impact your ability to safely and comfortably execute your plans to visit your daughter later that day.
- Another example based on the considerations listed above would be to include functional training exercises on the days you perform similar movements in the other components of your fitness routine. If you perform strength training for lower body muscles on a specific day, you could include your sit to stands, lunges, and floor transfers on that same day. This would help reinforce the movement patterns, provide more repetition for your body to accommodate to these activities, and will also improve your balance system.
    - A different theory would be to purposely include functional training exercises on the days where you train opposing muscle groups. For example, training your squats, lunges, and floor transfers on the days where you perform cardio and upper body strength training exercises. This may allow you to perform more repetitions and include more resistance or weight when performing your functional training since those specific muscle groups won't be as

fatigued as they would had you performed strength training beforehand.
- There is no "cookie cutter" way to include these exercises into your routine. The key is to be intentional and strategic, reassess, and then make adjustments as necessary.

Create a Supportive Environment

- Be realistic about your goals and your schedule. Set yourself up for success by planning and scheduling sufficient time to complete your routine and incorporate your functional training.
- Environment is important. Ensure your surroundings are safe and you have the appropriate space and equipment to execute your functional training exercises successfully.
- Always have stable surfaces around for upper extremity support if needed. Clear the floor around you so that if you have a near-fall or fall you minimize the risk of injury. Invest in knee pads or a padded mat for the floor if you are performing any high-risk movements, floor transfers, or exercises on the floor. Ask for supervision or assistance from family or friends if you feel unstable or unsafe when starting out specific movements. Ensure the temperature is appropriate and comfortable so that you can focus on your form, technique, and safety during your exercises.
- Take a second to plan, check off the items you'll need, and assess the environment you are working within prior to each session. Clean and sanitize yourself and

all equipment well after each session to prevent health complications.

Adding functional movements to your fitness routine is a game changer for staying independent and keeping fit. Finding specific ways to tailor your fitness routine to your abilities and long-term goals, while including these functional training exercises, is the key to living a custom-made ageless fitness lifestyle.

7.4 Improving Mobility and Range of Motion for Daily Tasks

Improving mobility and preserving full range of motion is an integral component of being able to maintain the freedom to choose to participate in any and every activity you choose as you age. The more mobility and range of motion you have, the more your body is able to safely and comfortably do without injury. This creates endless possibilities for you as an older adult, including being able to travel, engage in activities with your kids and grandkids, care for pets or your spouse if necessary, continue to work in your career, volunteer when you retire, etc. Making strides toward greater mobility will guarantee that you can keep on doing the things you love, no matter how challenging they may be. In addition to bolstering your autonomy, this lets you fully immerse yourself in the things you love doing in a care-free manner.

Improving your flexibility and mobility is about more than just being in shape--it is about being able to live life to the fullest.

You can overcome the typical difficulties that come with aging that might restrict your mobility by implementing the correct strategies and workouts. You can plan for better mobility and general well-being in your daily life by making these practices a part of your everyday routine. Improving your mobility and range of motion will equip you to confidently and gracefully tackle the obstacles of aging.

Here are aspects to focus on which target mobility and range of motion, and will result in a positive impact on your daily routine outside of your workouts if performed consistently :

Regular Stretching

- Perform stretching exercises regularly, ideally daily.
- Target major muscle groups, including legs, hips, back, shoulders, and neck.
- Incorporate dynamic movements for warm-ups and static stretches for cool downs.

Full Range of Motion (ROM) Exercises

- Perform exercises that promote a full range of motion in joints.
- Focus on the end-range or end-feel of a joint, and take 1-2 seconds to hold the exercise at the end of the range of motion in order to promote increased flexibility and ensure you are reaching full range of motion.

- Additional exercises to promote and focus specifically on full ROM that can be included are: leg swings, arm circles, and gentle joint rotations.

Joint Mobility Exercises

- Engage in exercises specifically designed to facilitate joint mobility.
- Some examples are: ankle circles, wrist rolls, and neck tilts.
- These can be performed throughout the day at your desk, or during sets of different exercises during your workout to provide relief and promote consistent joint flexibility/mobility.

Yoga and Tai Chi

- Both of these practices emphasize flowing movements that enhance flexibility, balance, and overall mobility.
- Incorporating these practices on an "active recovery" or rest day is a viable option for inclusion into your routine. You may also consider substituting balance exercises or functional training exercises one day and including either yoga or tai chi in your routine instead, since they have overlapping factors.
- Guidance while practicing is ideal and readily available online or in group fitness settings.

Aquatic Exercises

- Water provides resistance and also supports the body, making aquatic exercises especially gentle on the joints.
- Examples: water aerobics, swimming, leg lifts in the water.
- Exercising in the water is an excellent way to target painful or problematic areas (i.e.: areas with decreased range of motion or prior injury) since it supports, or unweights, the body compared to overground activity.
- For example, if you have a prior injury in your left knee and tend to favor the right knee when walking, you can focus on single leg standing on the left leg in the water, and slowly take away arm support, progressing to performing full range of motion knee bends either in standing or in sitting on a step while in the water. These exercises will be far less painful and uncomfortable if performed in the water compared to overground.

Foam Rolling and Self-Myofascial Release

- These techniques help relieve muscle tightness and improve flexibility.
- Gently roll over different muscle groups, focusing on areas of tension.
- Can be performed both before and after a workout, and as often as necessary.

Massage Therapy

- Helps relieve muscle tightness and tension; improves flexibility.
- Consider getting occasional professional massages.
- Learn self-massage techniques for daily maintenance.
- Focus on painful or problematic areas.
- Goal is to relieve tension and regain symmetry in postural muscles for recovery as well as preservation of good postural technique with mobility/repetitive movements.

Daily Movement

- Stay active. Even the days where you are not performing a scheduled workout, make it a point to decrease sedentary time.
- Break up long periods of sitting or lying in bed with breaks in standing and walking around.

Mobility and range of motion activities can easily be incorporated into your daily routine and become an automatic practice at certain points within your day. While they can and should be part of your fitness routine, it is extremely beneficial to find ways to include some of these practices in your daily routine outside of your workout. Changing a daily habit to include some of these exercises will afford increased joint health and ease of performance of daily tasks. Small changes over time make a big difference.

7.5 Enhancing Strength and Endurance for Independent Living

We've discussed the importance and the implementation process of strength and endurance training in older adulthood. Tying it together with functional training, specifically maintaining independence, in older adulthood is the ultimate goal. Being able to freely live an active fitness lifestyle of your choice, with little to no physical restrictions, and the knowledge to work around your abilities and limitations, is the key to long-lasting fulfillment as we age.

Strength training is an integral part of any exercise routine, and is especially important in older adulthood. It should be tailored to each individual, as discussed in previous chapters. Once you have established a sound strength training routine, and incorporate functional training exercises as well, you have laid the foundation for a stronger body that will provide you benefits in your everyday life. Depending on your personal goals, this newfound strength can continue to work in your favor to enhance your body's abilities. Living independently as long as possible is a goal for all adults as we age. It becomes increasingly difficult as we age and health complications arise. Once your ageless fitness program becomes a lifestyle, the habits you have created will sustain a stronger physically fit body, opening up doors and opportunities you may have never thought would be possible in your older years.

Endurance is equally important in order to provide the stamina required for a productive day. Regardless of the variability in demand each person's day may contain, there is no downfall to feeling like you can keep up with a productive day's worth of work, self-care, and social interaction. Living independently requires a certain amount of muscular and cardiovascular endurance just to simply take care of your own personal self-care needs. Not to mention keeping up with a house, and even a dependent family member such as an aging parent, spouse, or sick child. Consistency with your fitness routine provides the opportunity and option to not have to depend on anyone else. The more you take advantage of building your overall endurance, the more possibilities you have to not just live independently in your everyday life with your family, but also to enjoy what life has to offer above and beyond outside of that. For example, the more endurance you build, the easier activities such as traveling to new places, keeping up with your grandchildren, and going shopping at a new mall become.

A benefit to being stronger as you age is the ability to maintain the independence to dress yourself, bathe yourself, groom yourself, cook for yourself and your family, etc. However, the stronger and more independent you become, the possibilities of participating in more advanced tasks become a reality. Instrumental activities of daily living are considered more complex activities. These may be activities that you once required assistance with from family or friends, or even a hired person. Examples of these activities are: cooking a celebration meal for a retirement gathering or a traditional holiday, shopping all day in a large mall, managing finances for your household, using public transportation, or driving long distances. As you progress and settle into your ageless fitness lifestyle, reassess those more complicated daily tasks that you never thought you would be able to do, or that you felt like you were having difficulty maintaining, and notice how you may surprise yourself with newfound abilities.

Cognitive, emotional, and psychological independence are vital to being able to successfully and safely remain independent as we age. Retaining cognitive abilities to remember important information and make informed decisions is necessary in order to be able to live alone and partake in running a household. It is also important to be able to solve problems and navigate daily challenges. Achieving a sense of emotional well-being and resilience, maintaining a positive self-image and confidence, and coping with life changes and challenges are all a part of being able to function independently, as problems are inevitable and are likely to arise at various times and in various forms. Strength and endurance gained through consistent participation and progression in a fitness routine play a large role in mental and emotional acuity. Fitness level is undoubtedly correlated to mental and emotional independence in addition to physical independence.

Social independence is another benefit to enhancing strength and endurance and continually working on functional training. Maintaining relationships with family, friends, and community members provides loads of psychological benefits. Engaging in social activities, hobbies, and events can provide physical benefits which can occur inadvertently as one is distracted and participating in pleasurable activities such as playing games, attending community events, and socializing with other people. It is also gratifying to be able to be part of your community and contribute to it in various ways. This type of social interaction and involvement requires a certain level of physical capability that your ageless fitness lifestyle will provide.

Personal safety is another component to independent living that should be prioritized and taken very seriously. Being prepared for emergencies and knowing how to handle emergent situations at home, while driving, or while in public, are crucial to being able to safely live alone and travel into your community alone. Having an awareness of your surroundings and being able to react in situations that require you to make quick decisions in order to maintain personal safety or the safety of those around you, is essential. The combination of strength, endurance, and mental sharpness that an ageless fitness lifestyle provides facilitates one being able to remain calm and make decisions to keep themselves physically safe in multi-faceted situations and unknown circumstances.

Remaining consistent and even taking your fitness routine to the next level are vital to being able to live on your own, and lead a fulfilling life, as you get older. Allow these different factors of independence to serve as motivation for continuing to enhance your strength and endurance as you step into older adulthood.

CHAPTER 8

Posture Improvement and Back Pain Relief

8.1 Understanding the Impact of Aging on Posture and Back Health

Aging can have a significant impact on posture and back health due to various physiological changes that occur in the musculoskeletal system. Understanding these changes is crucial for adopting proactive measures to maintain good posture and back health as one ages. Here are some of the key ways in which aging can impact posture and back health:

Disc Degeneration

- Intervertebral discs, which act as cushions between the vertebrae, can undergo degenerative changes over time.
- Reduced disc height, decreased water content, and wear and tear can contribute to stiffness, decreased flexibility, and pain.

- Reduced disc height and water content can lead to decreased shock absorption and flexibility, influencing overall spinal alignment.

Loss of Bone Density (Osteoporosis)

- Aging is associated with a gradual loss of bone density, leading to conditions such as osteoporosis.
- Weakened vertebrae are more susceptible to fractures, which can cause back pain and affect overall spine stability. Weakened bones can also affect posture and movement patterns.

Changes in Spinal Joints

- Degenerative changes in the facet joints (small joints that connect vertebrae) can occur with age.
- Joint degeneration may lead to arthritis and inflammation, contributing to stiffness and pain in the back.
- Arthritis and inflammation in these joints may affect movement and contribute to changes in posture.

Muscle Atrophy and Weakness

- Aging is associated with a natural loss of muscle mass (sarcopenia) and strength.
- Weakened muscles may not provide adequate support for the spine, leading to instability, poor posture, and an increased risk of back pain.

Changes in Spinal Alignment

- With age, changes in spinal alignment may occur, such as a gradual loss of the natural curvature of the spine.
- Altered spinal alignment can contribute to muscle imbalances, increased pressure on certain structures, and the development of back pain.
- Loss of the natural curvature of the spine, such as increased thoracic kyphosis (rounded upper back), may lead to a stooped posture, affecting overall spinal alignment.

Reduced Elasticity of Connective Tissues

- Ligaments and tendons lose elasticity over time.
- Reduced flexibility of connective tissues may contribute to stiffness and limited range of motion in the spine.

Nerve Compression

- Conditions such as spinal stenosis, where the spinal canal narrows, become more prevalent with age.
- Narrowing of the spinal canal can lead to compression of nerves, causing pain, numbness, and tingling in the back and legs.

Muscle Imbalances

- As muscle strength and flexibility decline, postural imbalances may develop.

- Imbalances, such as tightness in certain muscle groups and weakness in others, can lead to poor posture and increased risk of back pain.

Reduced Joint Flexibility

- Aging can lead to gradual reduction in joint flexibility.
- Stiffness and decreased range of motion may influence posture and make it challenging to maintain proper alignment.

Disc Herniation

- Aging can make intervertebral discs more prone to herniation or bulging.
- Disc herniation can lead to compression of spinal nerves, causing back pain and radicular symptoms.
- These symptoms lead to movement compensations and as a result cause postural imbalances and asymmetries.

Aging can influence posture and back health through a combination of structural and functional changes. Adopting a proactive approach that includes regular exercise, ergonomic practices, and flexibility training can help mitigate the impact of aging and promote optimal posture and spinal health.

8.2 Assessing Posture and Identifying Areas of Improvement

Assessing posture involves observing the alignment of various body parts and identifying any deviations from the expected norm. A thorough posture assessment can provide valuable insights into musculoskeletal health, potential imbalances, and areas that may require attention.

Plumb Line Alignment

The "Plumb Line Alignment" is a postural assessment mentioned in Chapter 2 that is utilized to evaluate the alignment of various body segments in relation to a vertical line (plumb line) when a person is standing. This assessment provides insights into postural alignment and can help identify any deviations or asymmetries that may contribute to musculoskeletal issues or discomfort.

The individual is asked to stand comfortably in a relaxed, natural position, preferably barefoot. The assessment is conducted in front of a plumb line, which is a straight, vertical line, suspended from above. Specific anatomical landmarks and body segments are assessed for alignment with the plumb line. Common points include:

- Head: midpoint of the ear canal
- Shoulders: midpoint of the acromion processes
- Spine: midpoint between the shoulder blades
- Hips: midpoint of the iliac crests
- Knees: midpoint of the patella

- Ankles: midpoint of the lateral malleolus

The assessor visually observes the alignment of these points in relation to the plumb line from various perspectives, including the front, side, and possibly the back. You may use a mirror and visually assess yourself in relation to the plumb line as long as you are able to place yourself or the mirror in a location where you are able to maintain a neutral posture. Another option for self-assessment is to take a picture and/or video from each direction (front, side, back) using a timer and then analyze the footage. Deviations from the plumb line are noted, and any asymmetries or postural abnormalities are identified. Common deviations may include forward head posture, rounded shoulders, and pelvic tilt. Observations may be compared to expected norms and what "normal" posture should look like, where all landmarks are aligned with the plumb line. Key considerations to look for when analyzing your posture against the plumb line are :

- Forward head posture: determine if the head is positioned significantly forward relative to the rest of the body.
- Shoulder and pelvic alignment: assess whether one shoulder is higher than the other and if one side of the pelvis, or hip, is higher than the other.
- Spinal curves: observe whether there is an excessive curvature or flattening of the spine.
- Lower extremity alignment: observe alignment of knees and ankles in comparison to the plumb line and note any asymmetries.

The plumb line assessment can guide posture correction interventions. From these results, you learn what areas of the body to target for postural exercises to include in your fitness routine, and then select specific exercises for those areas. You can use the plumb line to reassess your progress and modify your exercises after a set amount of time of working on these areas (usually ~2-3 months, depending on the frequency of exercise).

Postural Assessment Forms

Postural assessment forms are tools used to systematically evaluate and document postural alignment of older adults. A postural assessment form includes sections for recording relevant anatomical landmarks and observations. Here is a general outline of what a postural assessment form for older adults might/should include:

General Appearance

- Stature: tall, average, short
- Body weight distribution: symmetrical or asymmetrical
- Overall posture: upright, stooped, or leaning

Head and Neck

- Head position: neutral, forward head, or tilted
- Chin position: level, elevated, or lowered
- Neck curvature: normal, increased, or decreased

Shoulders

- Height: symmetrical or asymmetrical
- Position: rounded or retracted (sitting back and upright)
- Shoulder blades: winged or set close together, symmetrical or asymmetrical

Pelvis (hip bone)

- Tilted forward or back?
- Alignment: symmetrical from one side to the other or asymmetrical
- Rotated in or out?

Legs

- Knee alignment: valgus (leaned in toward each other, "knock knees") or varus (leaned outward, "bow legged")
- Ankle alignment: pronation (weight on inside of foot), supination (weight on outside of foot), or neutral
- Foot arches: normal, flat, or high

Walking Analysis

- Walking pattern: smooth or regular
- Step length: short or long
- Foot placement: toe-in, toe-out, or neutral

Observations from Side View

- Alignment of ear, shoulder, hip, knee, and ankle

- Forward or backward lean of the trunk

Observations from Back View

- Alignment of spine, shoulders, and hips
- Notice any asymmetries from one side to the other

Using this form as a guide for noting asymmetries and aspects which fall outside of neutral, upright, posture will directly guide posture correction interventions. These forms can be used as an objective measure and guide for areas to target and exercises to select for your fitness routine. These forms can also be performed or reviewed by healthcare professionals, such as a physical therapist, if you are working with one. The idea is that you may use them in a self-guided fashion, or use them with a professional.

Digital Posture Analysis

The idea behind digital posture analysis is to leverage technology to provide a detailed and visual assessment of an individual's posture. These tools are designed to analyze body alignment, identify postural deviations, and offer insights to guide posture correction exercises. Different digital posture analysis tools generally share common features and can be used as self-guided postural assessment tools. Here is an overview of how digital posture analysis can be conducted for older adults :

Capture Images or Video

- Use a camera or smartphone to capture images or videos of yourself from different angles (front, sides, back).
- Use a dedicated app or software to upload and process the captured images or video.

Landmark Identification

- Use a software tool that uses algorithms to automatically identify key anatomical landmarks on the body, such as the head, shoulders, spine, hips, knees, and ankles.
- Algorithms on these tools can also analyze the alignment of identified landmarks in relation to established norms.
- Deviations from the expected alignment are identified, and the analysis compares your posture to ideal postural alignment.

Visual Feedback

- Results are often presented in visual formats, such as diagrams or graphs, showing your posture from different perspectives.
- Deviations or areas of concern may be color-coded for easy identification.

Advanced Options for Analysis and Intervention

- Some tools provide angle measurements to quantify the degree of deviation in specific body segments.

- Tools may offer interactive 3D models that allow you to rotate and zoom in on specific body segments which provide real-time feedback and recommendations for correcting posture.
- Some tools may allow for the comparison of posture over time, showing improvements or areas that require ongoing attention.
- There are also options that integrate with electronic health record systems for seamless collaboration with healthcare providers.
- Tools may offer personalized recommendations for exercises or interventions based on identified postural issues.
- Information materials on proper ergonomics and posture may be provided.

There are various options for digital posture analysis tools that exist in our current technology-driven society. These tools can be found on smartphone apps, and can serve as a user-friendly, self-guided option for older adults to assess posture and identify areas of improvement. It is always recommended to do your research on the different features of these tools in order to ensure that you are selecting a resource that is most appropriate and fitting for your body and technological preferences. Some examples of these digital posture analysis tools for your reference are: Upright GO, PostureScreen Mobile, BioSensics' Gait Keeper, Aline, Perfect Posture Workout, Lumo Lift, SquatScreen, Posture Corrector—Straighten Your Back at Home, and PhysiApp. Digital posture analysis tools can be beneficial for providing objective data, visual feedback, remote accessibility, progress tracking, educational support, and integration with healthcare providers.

Assessing your posture and identifying areas of improvement is a proactive step in committing to a pain-free ageless fitness lifestyle. Once you have identified areas of improvement, it is essential to incorporate posture-correcting exercises into your fitness routine.

8.3 Incorporating Posture-Correcting

Posture correcting exercises for older adults focus on strengthening key muscles, improving flexibility, and promoting overall body awareness. Incorporating these exercises into your routine can contribute to better posture and reduced discomfort. The beauty of posture correcting exercises is that they can be done as part of your workout routine, your daily routine, or both. Building these exercises into your rest breaks while working or watching television can facilitate these movements becoming a seamless part of your daily routine, and is absolutely doable. These types of exercises promote optimal posture which leads to overall improvement with mobility and decreased pain. Therefore, practicing them as much as possible is recommended. When integrating these exercises into your life, it is most favorable to incorporate them into your daily routine as well as your fitness routine, if at all possible.

Below are some effective posture-correcting exercises for older adults. Visit your supplemental material guide at https://bit.ly/3x3FmbJ for videos of these exercises.

Chin Tucks

- Strengthens the muscles at the back of the neck, helping to counteract forward head posture.
    - Sit or stand with a straight spine. Can also be performed while lying on your back in bed.
    - Gently tuck your chin towards your chest without tilting your head.

Shoulder Blade Squeezes

- Targets the muscles between the shoulder blades, promoting better upper back posture.
    - Sit or stand with a straight back. Can be performed lying on your back as well
    - Squeeze your shoulder blades together as if trying to hold a pencil between them.

Shoulder Rolls

- Improves flexibility and mobility in the shoulders and upper back and counteracts rounded shoulders.
    - Sit or stand tall, arms relaxed at your sides.
    - Slowly roll your shoulders backwards in a circular motion.

- Keep your chest open and your spine elongated. Squeeze your shoulder blades together and down as you roll your shoulders back.

Thoracic Extension Exercise

- Improves mobility in the upper back and counteracts rounded shoulders.
  - Sit on a stability ball or chair with your back straight.
  - Place your hands behind your head.
  - Gently arch your upper back, extending through the thoracic spine.

Wall Angels

- Strengthens the muscles around the shoulder blades and promotes better posture.
  - Stand with your back against a wall.
  - Bring your arms up to shoulder height, elbows bent at 90 degrees. Keep your arms and forearms up against the wall.
  - Slide your arms up the wall, keeping your elbows and wrists in contact with the wall. Squeeze your shoulder blades together and down on as your arms slide down the wall.

Perform each exercise for several repetitions. Start with 1 set of 10 repetitions, and increase sets as you feel comfortable. It is beneficial to perform a high number of repetitions with this type of exercise. As long as you do not feel pain or discomfort while performing the exercise, it is safe to increase repetitions and sets. Focus on slow, controlled movements with correct form and body awareness while performing these exercises. Mindfulness of body alignment during these exercises translates into mindfulness of body alignment during daily tasks, which leads to achievement of the overall goal—improved posture.

8.4 Strengthening Core Muscles for Better Posture

Core exercises play a crucial role in improving posture, especially for older adults. A strong core helps support the spine, maintain proper alignment, and reduce the risk of musculoskeletal issues. The muscles in your abdomen, low back, and pelvis are foundational for supporting and stabilizing the spine. Strengthening them improves posture and helps alleviate back strain and pain.

Outlined below are core exercises that contribute to better posture in older adults. For video demonstration of these exercises, visit your supplemental material resource at https://bit.ly/3x3FmbJ.

Pelvic Tilts

- Engages the lower abdominal muscles and helps improve pelvic alignment.
    - Lie on your back with knees bent and feet flat on the floor.

o Tighten your abdominal muscles to flatten your lower back against the floor.

Elbow Plank

- Strengthens the core muscles, including the abdominal and back muscles.
  o Start in a forearm plank position with elbows under shoulders.
  o Keep your body in a straight line from head to heels, engaging your core.

Dead Bug Exercise

- Targets the deep core muscles, promoting stability.
  o Lie on your back with arms extended toward the ceiling and legs lifted.
  o Lower one arm and the opposite leg toward the floor, while keeping the lower back pressed into the floor.
  o Return to the starting position and repeat with the other arm and leg.

Bird-Dog Exercise

- Strengthens the core and back muscles, promotes thoracic extension.
  o Start on hands and knees in a tabletop position.
  o Extend one arm forward and the opposite leg backward.
  o Hold for a few seconds and then return to the starting position. Repeat with the other arm and leg.

Bridge

- Strengthens the glutes, hamstrings, and lower back, promoting stability in the pelvic region.
    - Lie on your back with knees bent and feet hip-width apart.
    - Lift your hips toward the ceiling, forming a straight line from shoulders to knees.
    - Hold for a few seconds, then lower back down.

Superman

- Strengthens the glutes and back muscles, promotes extension in the spine.
    - Lie on your stomach with arms extended in front of you. Lift your arms, chest, and legs off the ground, engaging your back and core muscles.

Some of these exercises may overlap with the core exercises in your fitness routine due to their multi-faceted nature. These exercises help promote better posture, but are also excellent for general core strengthening as well as stability, which inadvertently improves balance. While performing these exercises, focus on maintaining proper form and breathe steadily. This will help you engage your core muscles and prevents strain on other muscles. Incorporate these exercises into your routine regularly for optimal benefits--either on a core strengthening segment/day or on a separate posture-correcting segment/day.

8.5 Stretching and Mobility Exercises

Experiencing back pain and discomfort as you age is common, but it doesn't have to be a permanent part of your life. Integrating stretching and mobility exercises into your daily routine can significantly alleviate, and even prevent, back pain. These exercises also facilitate improved posture through recruitment of the trunk and pelvic muscles during movements that promote optimal positioning and alignment of the spine. Stretching and mobility exercises targeted at improving posture and alleviating back pain help increase flexibility, reduce muscle tightness, and enhance overall mobility.

Specific stretching and mobility exercises recommended for older adults to promote better posture and decrease back pain are discussed below. Video demonstration of these exercises can be found in your supplemental material resource, at https://bit.ly/3x3FmbJ.

Child's Pose

- Start on hands and knees in a tabletop position.
- Sit back on your heels, extending your arms forward.

Cat-Camel Exercise

- Start on hands and knees in a tabletop position.
- Alternate between arching your back upwards and dipping it down towards the floor.

Seated Twist

- Sit in a chair with your back straight.
- Twist your torso to one side, holding the back of the chair.
- Hold 30 seconds, then twist to the other side.

Shoulder Circles

- In standing or sitting, extend your arms out to the side, keeping your elbows straight.
- Roll your shoulders forward, rotating your arms in a forward motion, making small circles. Gradually increase the size of the circles.
- Alternate directions, rolling your shoulders backward, making small, then gradually bigger circles.
- Alternate arms.

Hip Circles

- In standing position, move your hips up then out to the side and back, in a circular motion. Alternate legs.

Ankle Alphabet

- In a comfortable seated position, rotate your ankle in all directions, as if you were writing the alphabet in the air with your foot. Alternate legs.

POSTURE IMPROVEMENT AND BACK PAIN RELIEF

Performing these exercises consistently throughout the day, as well as either before or after your workout routine, will result in increased comfort with mobility in your daily life.

CONCLUSION

Maintaining an Ageless Fitness Lifestyle

Making fitness and wellness a priority in your life is an investment in your health in every way. Not only is regular exercise important for your physical health, but it is also important for your mental and emotional well-being. This regularity is imperative in order to gracefully, comfortably, and actively age. It is necessary to maintain strength, improve your flexibility, and keep your balance. Being able to live on your own and have a fulfilling, satisfying life in older adulthood is directly correlated to the work you put in towards your fitness and wellness goals.

Adapting to Your Evolving Needs

Your body naturally goes through changes as you go through different stages of life. Because of this evolution, you need to be proactive and flexible with your exercise routine. Not only is recognizing and understanding these changes a sign of wisdom, it is also important for your health. It means realizing that what worked for you in the past might not work as well or fit your current needs.

Your body's evolvement means that picking the right type of workouts is crucial. For example, cardio exercises with less force become a better choice. These exercises, like swimming, walking, or riding a bike, are good for your heart without putting too much stress on your joints. These kinds of workouts are very important for keeping your heart healthy while also taking into account the natural considerations that come with getting older.

In addition, strength training changes in a new way. You do not have to lift the heaviest weights anymore. Instead, you should do an exercise that makes you stronger while keeping your joints safe. The focus changes to exercises that make your muscles stronger and more stable without putting too much stress on your body. Exercises that improve your balance and stability are also very important and should be a part of your practice. Falls can become a legitimate concern as you get older, and these are very important for lowering your risk and keeping you safe as you navigate your daily life. Adding tai chi, yoga, and balance drills to your routine can make a big difference in how stable you feel and how confident you feel.

The goal is to stay committed to your health at every age by changing your workout routine to fit your evolving needs. To adapt, you need to pay attention to your body's signs and be ready to change the way you work out based on what your body is telling you in every moment. To stay healthy, it is important to find a balance between pushing your body to grow and staying within its limits. With this approach, you build an effective fitness plan that is sustainable over time.

Holistic Approach to Fitness

As an older adult, it is vital to take a comprehensive approach to fitness. This is a path that includes more than just working out. It includes nutrition, mental agility, and community fellowship. This well-rounded method maintains physical health as well as mental and emotional health, which are integral parts of living a happy life in older adulthood.

Eating healthy, well-balanced nutritious meals is the basis for this all-around approach. This means giving your body foods that are both healthy and good for your changing dietary needs. It is advised to focus on healthy fats, lean proteins, whole grains, fruits, vegetables, and energy-dense foods. These foods facilitate keeping your body healthy and provide the energy required to participate in your fitness routine.

Along with nutrition, mental health is very critical. Just like working out your body, keeping your mind positively stimulated and in a good state is imperative. There are many approaches and habits that can facilitate this, such as completing puzzles, reading, learning something new, taking a class, meditating, joining a book club, or simply having intentional and deep talks with family and friends. These activities can help keep your brain sharp and slow down cognitive loss, which can be a worry for many people as they get older.

There can be many barriers that make it hard to stay fit as you get older. You have to be strong and ready to change to make it through the journey. This means being able to change your exercise plan if your health changes, or searching for new activities or interests that make you feel happy and motivated. With a positive and proactive attitude, you are facing these difficulties in a way that will lead to inevitable success and inner peace.

Making small changes, such as modifying the intensity of your workouts or adding more rest days, are examples of this mindset and approach. On other occasions, bigger changes may be warranted, like finding new ways to exercise if the old ones get too hard or painful. The key is to pay attention to your body, treat it with kindness and grace, and make sure that the things you do are in line with what your body can and needs in every moment.

Starting this exercise journey does not have to be something you do by yourself. The support of a group, such as in a local exercise class, an online community, or the company of friends and family, can make your experience more enjoyable. Not only do these networks offer useful help, like exercise or food tips, but they also offer emotional support by providing a place to talk about goals, wins, struggles, and words of support and encouragement.

In these groups, whether they are in person or online, you will find people who are going through similar life experiences and changes. Sharing stories and advice, acknowledging each other's successes, and being there for each other when things get tough, are all things that keep people united and motivated. They remind you that even though your process is unique, everyone has been through something relatable, and that support is always near.

In the end, living a fit lifestyle is not age-dependent and is a journey of constant growth. It is about accepting each part of your health—physical, mental, and emotional—and having fun throughout the process. Every time you take a step, like trying a new recipe, picking up a new skill, or taking a community class, you are not only working towards your fitness, but you are also making new connections and incorporating pleasurable activities. With this all-around method, you can ensure that your older adult years will be not only lived, but also enjoyed--filled with health, happiness, and endless joy.

Living the Ageless Fitness Philosophy Daily

The concept of ageless fitness transcends the conventional notion of exercise. It's a lifelong journey, an evolving process that intertwines with the ever-changing tapestry of life. As you grow older, it's essential to remain actively receptive to new knowledge and breakthroughs in health and wellness. The fitness world is continually advancing, with fresh research, innovative workout trends, and updated health recommendations emerging regularly. Staying informed and adjusting your routine in response to these developments ensures that your approach to fitness remains dynamic.

Ageless fitness is a philosophy, a mindset that promotes a holistic, active, and joyous lifestyle at any age. It's not confined to the parameters of a gym or a fitness class—the goal is for it to be a part of your everyday life. This philosophy encourages you to embrace change gracefully, understand and respect your body's evolving capabilities, and find pleasure and satisfaction in staying active. It's about recognizing that every movement, every activity – whether it's a morning walk, gardening, dancing, or yoga – contributes to your overall vitality and engagement with life and your surroundings.

As you turn the last page of this guide to ageless fitness, consider it not an end but a milestone in your ongoing journey. Each day is a fresh canvas, an opportunity to reinforce your physical strength, stimulate your mind, and uplift your spirit. Your commitment to this journey is a commitment to yourself – to live vibrantly, with a positive outlook, and a spirit that soars well into your years of older adulthood.

Your pursuit of an ageless fitness lifestyle is an everlasting journey, one that evolves and grows with you over the years. It's about consistently finding balance and harmony in your physical activities, nutritional choices, and mental health practices. Remember, the journey to ageless fitness is as much about nurturing the soul as it is about conditioning the body.

It's about celebrating each step, acknowledging your progress, and always looking forward to what lies ahead.

As you embark on each new day, do so with the intention to enhance your physical, mental, and emotional well-being. Keep moving, exploring, and experiencing the joys of life in all of its fullness. Let this journey of ageless fitness be a testament to your resilience, a celebration of your strength, and a path to a life of fulfillment and joy. Here's to aging not just with grace, but with energy, enthusiasm, and an evergreen spirit of adventure!

www.ingramcontent.com/pod-product-compliance
Lightning Source LLC
Chambersburg PA
CBHW060948050426
42337CB00052B/1715